Learning the Language of Dentistry

Studies in Corpus Linguistics (SCL)

ISSN 1388-0373

SCL focuses on the use of corpora throughout language study, the development of a quantitative approach to linguistics, the design and use of new tools for processing language texts, and the theoretical implications of a data-rich discipline.

For an overview of all books published in this series, please see
http://benjamins.com/catalog/scl

Volume 93

Learning the Language of Dentistry
Disciplinary corpora in the teaching of English for Specific Academic Purposes
by Peter Crosthwaite and Lisa Cheung

Learning the Language of Dentistry

Disciplinary corpora in the teaching of English for Specific Academic Purposes

Peter Crosthwaite
University of Queensland

Lisa Cheung
The University of Hong Kong

John Benjamins Publishing Company
Amsterdam / Philadelphia

The paper used in this publication meets the minimum requirements of the American National Standard for Information Sciences – Permanence of Paper for Printed Library Materials, ANSI z39.48-1984.

Cover design: Françoise Berserik
Cover illustration from original painting *Random Order*
by Lorenzo Pezzatini, Florence, 1996.

DOI 10.1075/scl.93

Cataloging-in-Publication Data available from Library of Congress:

ISBN 978 90 272 0427 1 (HB)
ISBN 978 90 272 6198 4 (E-BOOK)

John Benjamins Publishing Company · https://benjamins.com

Table of contents

Acknowledgements

This book could not have been possible without the assistance of a great number of colleagues, support staff and family. We would first and foremost like to thank Prof. Ken Hyland for spearheading the English-in-the-Discipline movement at the University of Hong Kong, creating the context in which this entire study was conceived and created, as well as for providing the foreword to this volume. Next, we would like to thank Prof. Ricky Kwok, Victor Y. L. Wong and Tyrone Kwok of the HKU Technology-Enhanced Learning Initiative (TELI) at HKU, who assisted us in creating the innovative corpus platform involved in this study, as well as Dr. Lillian Wong, who was the leader of the Teacher Development Grant project on a HKU Graduate Corpus that helped bring the Centre for Applied English Studies and TELI together on corpus-related projects. We would also like to thank Joyce Oiwun Cheung for assisting greatly with analysis of the learner analytic data that formed the findings of Chapter 6, and wish her well in her Ph.D. studies. We extend our thanks to Prof. Thomas Flemming and Prof. Colman McGrath of the HKU Dentistry Faculty for their continued support and assistance throughout this project, as well the two ESAP teachers who provided interview data for Chapter 7. We are very grateful for the support and assistance of Jason Kessler, who provided detailed instructions and advice on his wonderful *Scattertext* tool, as well as Kristopher Kyle, who gratefully provided the wordlists used for his *SEANCE* tool, Laurence Anthony for *AntConc*, Andrea Nini for the *MAT tagger*, Gero Kunter for *Coquery*, Paul Rayson for *Wmatrix*, and other researchers whose corpus applications have made this type of research much easier than it used to be! We also thank Mia Yunmi Cho, and Erin and William Crosthwaite for their help and support during the writing process. Finally, thanks to God's faithful and unfailing love during this long research journey, and the late Peter Cheung for his enduring love and trust.

Foreword

Corpora and specialised English in the university curriculum

Ken Hyland
University of East Anglia

One of the most momentous decisions facing English teachers is the kind of language they should teach. At university this often boils down to following an English for General Academic Purposes (EGAP) approach, where teachers attempt to isolate the skills, language forms, and study activities thought to be common to all disciplines, or to seriously engage with the particular target language features their students most urgently need. The course described in this book takes the second path, taking the idea of specificity seriously in English language teaching. The course is the outcome of a particular set of circumstances in Hong Kong which involved the radical restructuring of the entire secondary and tertiary education systems and which provided an opportunity for us to completely rethink our provision of English to students at Hong Kong University.

As the unit responsible for English language teaching at HKU we were fortunate, at the time, to have the support of a forward-thinking Pro-vice chancellor, a considerable amount of autonomy and a group of committed teachers. As a consequence, we were able to respond to the curriculum changes by completely rewriting our entire undergraduate courses to offer students more context-sensitive forms of instruction based on closer cooperation with academic disciplines and research-informed course designs.

What sets English for academic purposes (EAP) apart from general language study is its focus on specific, purposeful uses of language. This is a 'context-reduced' variety which tends to be abstract, and less reliant on an immediate context for its coherence than the language of everyday interaction. But while the notion of specificity is at the heart of most definitions of EAP, debates continue over just how specific its purposes should be, and this influences both research and instruction (e.g. Hyland, 2016). The courses we designed were based on recognising that academic literacy in English presents a serious obstacle to many learners and is very different to the English they have learnt at school. Our new curriculum therefore determined that all undergraduates would take two English courses:

1. An EGAP course to all first-year students called 'Core University English' (CUE)
2. A more disciplinary specific 'English in the Discipline' (ED) course in later years.

Both types of course presented their own difficulties. CUE is designed to bridge the gap between the largely traditional grammar-focused, exam-oriented English familiar to the students from their secondary schools and the communicative expectations of disciplinary study. Making a virtue of heterogeneity, classes are deliberately composed of students from different faculties and draw on content from their common core courses to develop an understanding of spoken and written texts. There are obviously difficulties in identifying a 'core' in the language used across the university. Nesi and Gardner's (2011) corpus study of writing in UK universities, for example, distinguishes thirteen "genre families", ranging from research reports to empathy writing, which differ enormously in their social purposes, generic stages and preferred patterns of language. This EGAP course therefore sought to help students to structure coherent arguments, to show how they can present a stance through hedging and various kinds of evidence, to develop critical reading skills by identifying how an author's opinions are expressed, and to gain control over features like nominalisation, impersonality and lexical density.

Perhaps more challenging, however, was creating the ED courses because these had to incorporate the fact that the conventions of academic communication differ considerably across disciplines. The ability to comprehend and construct disciplinary arguments is at the heart of a conceptual understanding of a field, so that students must learn to craft their writing in community-specific ways. Language is tied to disciplines because it is inseparable from how we understand the world, and has a powerful influence on how students understand and engage with their disciplines because it reflects particular social practices and epistemologies. This famous quote from Bartholomae captures this perfectly:

> Every time a student sits down to write for us, he has to invent the university for the occasion – invent the university, that is, or a branch of it, like history, anthropology or economics or English. He has to learn to speak our language, to speak as we do, to try on the peculiar ways of knowing, selecting, evaluating, reporting, concluding, and arguing that define the discourse of our community.
>
> (Bartholomae, 1986: p. 4)

These "ways of knowing" are not learned by mastering grammar rules but by writing, so that learning a subject needs to be closely linked with learning to write a subject.

Learners, then, are required to think their way into their disciplines through writing, and identifying the particular language features, discourse practices, and communicative skills of target groups is a key part of curriculum design. Our conception of "English in the discipline" attempted to be sensitive to the considerable communicative demands which higher education places on students and acknowledge that their difficulties with English is not a linguistic deficit which can be topped up in a few language classes. Instead, it accepts that students have to take on new roles and engage with knowledge in new ways when they enter university. English in the Discipline, then, is our attempt to equip students with the communicative skills they need to participate in particular disciplinary contexts.

The creation of the ED courses therefore involved teachers in conducting investigative projects into the literacy demands and expectations of courses in different faculties and exploring new ways of delivering classes and monitoring progress. This involved, where possible, working in close collaboration with individual faculties and departments to ensure that the English courses aligned with the work students would do in their content courses. It also involved finding ways to offer students the means to extend their learning experience beyond the classroom. Language corpora proved a central resource in seeking to achieve both these goals: providing information on how students used language that was highly regarded by their professors, and as a means of encouraging students to use their considerable analytical skills to explore these uses.

The dentistry course therefore exploits two key aspects of corpora. On one hand they provided teachers and students with robust sources of target language, giving students access to naturally occurring, authentic data instead of invented examples. On the other hand, they contributed to a shift from teaching as imparting knowledge to teaching as mediating learning, allowing students to take a more active and reflective part in their learning.

In sum, the ED dentistry course discussed by my colleagues in this book explicitly rejects the idea that university English teaching involves beefing up generic language skills and shows how corpora can help students towards developing a new kind of literacy. It puts the concept of *specificity* at the heart of language instruction and supports student towards control of the discourses that their tutors and other disciplinary insiders are likely to find effective. I am certain that our efforts to implement English in the Discipline would have been far less successful without the assistance of corpus descriptions of language and a DDL approach to instruction.

References

Bartholomae, D. (1986). Inventing the university. *Journal of Basic Writing*, 5, 4–23.

Hyland, K. (2016). General and specific EAP. In K. Hyland & P. Shaw (Eds.), *Routledge handbook of EAP* (pp. 17–29). London: Routledge.

Nesi, H., & Gardner, S. (2011). *Genres across the disciplines. Student writing in Higher education.* Cambridge: Cambridge University Press.

CHAPTER 1

Getting to the 'root' of the problem

Introduction to the volume

1.1 EAP, EGAP, ESAP, and the ESAP conundrum for non-specialist disciplinary language tutors

This volume deals with the creation and analysis of specialised language corpora spanning three key genres of the dentistry discipline to gain a data-driven insight into the key lexico-grammatical features constitutive of the 'language of dentistry'. These findings were then used for the implementation of a new corpus-based data-driven learning pedagogy within a tertiary English for Specific Academic Purposes (ESAP) disciplinary writing programme for dentistry. The motivation for this volume was borne of a real, practical (and somewhat typical) conundrum encountered by its authors, who were tasked with redesigning the aforementioned undergraduate dentistry ESAP course at the world's top-ranked dentistry faculty within the University of Hong Kong. This chapter describes this conundrum in more detail, before outlining the means we employed to solve it.

ESAP refers to second language (L2)-specific training in disciplinary academic discourses, as opposed to English for General Academic Purposes (EGAP, Blue, 1988; Flowerdew, 2016). From a teaching perspective, this approach "targets the current and/or future academic or occupational needs of learners, focuses on the necessary language, genres, and skills to address these needs, and assists learners in meeting these needs through the use of general and/or discipline-specific teaching materials and methods" (Anthony, 2018: p. 1). Both ESAP and EGAP fall under the broader umbrella of English for Academic Purposes (EAP), itself a specialism within the field of English for Specific Purposes (ESP) (Hyland & Hamp-Lyons, 2002).[1] With English "undisputedly" the *lingua franca* of research and tertiary academic instruction, even in contexts where English is not widely spoken (Flowerdew, 2016: p. 6), there has been a significant global increase in the demand for EAP provision across the early months and years of university.

1. To explain further, ESAP is narrower in scope than is covered by the broader field of ESP, which may not necessarily involve academic discourse.

The vast majority of this instruction focuses on academic writing, which plays a gatekeeping role in determining eventual success or failure within the academy (Flowerdew, 2016), as well as entry into professional organisations and societies, and the facilitation of international collaboration (Morse & Nakahara, 2001). In the transition from secondary/high school to university, even students for whom English is a native or dominant language must quickly adapt to new expectations of academic literacy, alongside changes to their identity as writers (Christie, Tett, Cree, Hounsell & McCune, 2008; Nesi & Gardner, 2012). For students with English as an additional, weaker language, their competence in academic literacies both oral, and particularly written (Morrison & Evans, 2018) is confounded by a lack of knowledge about academic discourse on one hand, and the typical inaccuracy, inconsistency and incoherence of L2 production on the other (Morrison, 2014).

In the context of the present study, Hong Kong, English is the tertiary medium of instruction despite 75% of secondary schools operating with Cantonese as the preferred medium (Poon, 2010). A range of survey studies (e.g. Evans & Green, 2007; Evans & Morrison, 2011; Morrison 2014) have found Hong Kong undergraduates experience severe difficulties understanding lectures, acquiring technical vocabulary, and conforming to an academic register. Hyland (2016a: p. 240) goes as far to suggest that the students arriving at university "think they have landed on Mars", with academic writing in particular seen as "an alien form of literacy" (*ibid*). Within this context, the goal of EAP is therefore that of "demystifying academic discourses" (Hyland & Hamp-Lyons, 2002: p. 9), as well as confronting L2-specific deficiencies at the local and (particularly) global levels of written production.

In contexts where EAP instruction is offered, freshman undergraduate L2 students most commonly take courses in EGAP. In many cases, that is both the beginning and the end of their EAP training (Flowerdew, 2016). However, EGAP as an enterprise has frequently suffered from a perceived "disconnect" noticed by students between the kind of generic content and writing tasks assigned by EGAP instructors and the discipline-specific language demands of their subject majors (Hardy & Friginal, 2016: p. 119). Students' language needs within higher education (particular in the Hong Kong context) are "often centered around the question of [discipline] *specificity*" (Evans & Morrison, 2011: p. 206). While EGAP is itself a specific form of English instruction, those within the field have not yet reached a consensus over "just how specific its purposes should be" (Hyland, 2016b: p. 41). By the end of their first year of undergraduate studies, many students still lack awareness of the epistemologies and values of the discipline of which they are to eventually become a member (Hyland & Tse, 2009), and require further instruction in the discipline-specific language conventions of their target discourse community (Swales, 1990) or community of practice (Lave & Wenger, 1991). The notion that graduating students should be generally proficient in the discourses of the discipline they are to join is a key step in generating employable graduates, as shown in the following quote from a professional builder that summarises the expectations for vocational students intending to enter the construction industry:

> I reckon, like, you know, you look like a builder, you walk like a builder, you might as well talk like a builder, you know what I mean, and that way we can have a conversation, we can get into the conversation, how builders talk. Builders have their own sort of language. (Parkinson, Demecheleer & Mackay, 2017: p. 29)

Addressing how to learn this "own sort of language", EAP writing instruction (ideally) involves elements of what are known as 'learning-to-write' and 'writing-to-learn' (Manchón, 2011). The former involves a focus on the writer and the writing process, and includes instruction in planning, drafting and revising a text, instruction in the linguistic features of the text itself, and a focus on how the reader may respond to the text (Hirvela, Hyland & Manchón, 2016). The concept of 'writing-to-learn' can be subdivided into 'writing to learn content' and 'writing to learn language'. 'Writing to learn language' involves a specific focus on L2 development, typically measured through the improvement of accuracy, fluency or complexity (Cumming, 1990; Polio & Park, 2016). Development along these criteria is typically addressed in EGAP via direct written corrective feedback or through supplemental online 'grammar' or 'vocabulary' modules. 'Writing to learn content' within generic EGAP provision involves the acquisition of key writing skills including paraphrasing, finding sources, constructing a stance, etc., with the aim that students later 'transfer' (James, 2010, 2012) these skills to their disciplinary courses.

As mentioned, in many institutions, once undergraduate students have completed their EGAP obligations in the first semester or year of studies, they are (generally) left to fend for themselves when acquiring the specific disciplinary discourses of their subject majors. However, whether and how students eventually achieve this, and whether and why some students might be better than their peers at doing so is still a relatively underexplored phenomenon (Flowerdew & Costley, 2017). What we *do* know is that despite disciplinary writing "being at the heart of conceptual understanding of a field" (Hyland, 2013a: p. 241), there is a general lack of post-EGAP input from disciplinary tutors regarding the acquisition of disciplinary discourses. This is an issue made more difficult by disciplinary tutors' lack of expertise in resolving language problems, or unwillingness to resolve such problems, as exemplified in the following quote from a disciplinary tutor from the engineering discipline:

> If they have problems with language errors, that means they are not working hard enough. They are 21 years old. I mean, they should have a high level of ability already, not just what they have learnt since coming here. When I assess their writing I have to treat everybody equally so I grade grammar less, a very small percentage, maybe 5%. If we focus on the content, that puts everybody on the same playing field. (Hyland, 2013a: p. 245)

Worse still, disciplinary students are often unwilling to consult their disciplinary tutors regarding any language issue they may be facing, as exemplified in this quote from a student of social administration after receiving their disciplinary tutor's comments on their work:

> No. No advice on writing. Even if I ask, I think he [the disciplinary tutor] won't teach me much. I write it out myself by looking at the previous report samples and then put in the content. I believe he doesn't think it is difficult to write.
> (Hyland, 2013b: p. 183)

Disciplinary tutors often fail to realise that in successfully acquiring disciplinary discourses, students are acquiring the 'habitus', or identity and agency that characterise their chosen profession and distinguish it from others (Schryer, Lingard & Spafford, 2003). It is through this process that students eventually become enculturated into the profession before contributing to that discipline in the future through publication. It is under these difficult conditions that ESAP professionals attempt to develop the oral and written communication skills of their students in line with disciplinary expectations beyond freshman EGAP provision, becoming directly involved with ensuring students acquire the specificity so important to students' knowledge of their target discipline and their identity within it.

Having outlined the need for ESAP, we remind the reader here about the ESAP 'conundrum' that led to the creation of this volume. Put simply, the problem was that while the authors were responsible for the development of ESAP provision for students within the dentistry discipline, neither author happens to be, ever has been, nor plans to be a practicing dentist. We had never taken any training in dental procedures or clinical practice, and – to be perfectly honest – had not even read a single full dental research paper or article from any other key dentistry-related genre prior to the research undertaken in this volume. Yet, the task at hand was to re-develop, package and *sell* a disciplinary ESAP course to the university's dentistry faculty, aiming at developing students' awareness of the register and genres of dentistry writing while enculturating these students into their discipline.

Developing disciplinary language courses with only minimal subject knowledge is commonplace in ESAP. Despite being responsible for teaching students who are presumably already legitimate peripheral participants (Lave & Wenger, 1991) in their chosen discipline, ESAP tutors are – in almost all cases – not subject experts in fields outside of languages (although we are quite a diverse collective). Hutchinson and Waters (1987: p. 158) have characterised ESAP tutors as "reluctant dwellers in a strange and uncharted land", and ESAP professionals have been found to experience a "subject-knowledge dilemma" (Wu & Badger, 2009: p. 20) when devising courses and when dealing with disciplinary areas of knowledge they are unfamiliar with in classroom situations. To overcome this, ESAP tutors need to quickly gain knowledge of disciplinary cultures and values, knowledge of the epistemological basis of different disciplines, and knowledge of disciplinary genres and discourses (Ferguson, 1997: p. 85). In other words, ESAP tutors need to "investigate the specific epistemology, language, and practices of the target discipline and its community of practice, perhaps, themselves contributing to the research literature" (Flowerdew, 2016: p. 10).

This was a challenge that we, the authors, were willing to take on. But where to begin? How might an ESAP teacher with no specialist knowledge of the dentistry discipline reveal the discursive practices of dentistry in order to eventually teach such practices to future dentists? Here, we should probably mention that the two authors of this volume are not only ESAP professionals – they are also *corpus linguists* – and it is through the lens of corpora that the ESAP conundrum was to be solved.

In the remainder of this introduction, we now lay the foundations for the rationale and content of the empirical studies contained within this volume. This book is comprised of two major sections, each containing three chapters. Section 1 deals with a range of corpus analyses of texts spanning three key genres of the dentistry discipline, namely experimental research articles, case reports, and student/professional research reports within the field of Dental Public Health. Section 2 deals with how the results of the analyses conducted in Section 1 were used to generate teaching and learning materials and corpus-based pedagogical innovations within a dental ESAP programme before evaluating the impact of these innovations and outlining areas for future research.

1.2 Introduction to Section 1

In order to investigate the language and practices of the target discipline, one has to become familiar with the register of that discipline, determine whether there are any key genres particularly associated with that register, then analyse texts representative of these genres to derive the language features of the register. We can then induce from these features the discursive and identity-forming practices of the discipline, which, once made explicit, can then be taught to disciplinary students. The first section of this volume is devoted to how we achieved these goals through the creation and analysis of disciplinary corpora spanning three key genres of the dentistry discipline.

1.2.1 Definitions of register/genre

The original sense of register is that taken from music (Schubert, 2016). Register in linguistics is therefore "seen to be regulated in the same way as the musical tuning of an organ" (Dittmar, 2010, c.f. Schubert, 2016: p. 3). Taking this analogy further, Schubert suggests that competent language users are able to "fine-tune their linguistic choices according to their intended contextual functions" (p. 3). The role of the ESAP professional can therefore be seen as that of a conductor whose job it is to lead their novice orchestra through a concerto, ensuring that the sheet music – or register – provided to the band represents the piece they are to eventually play. The common problem with this situation, as we have described, is that the conductor is often just as much in the dark as the band about how to play the right tune.

There have been both 'narrow' and 'wide' approaches to the analysis of register from different sub-fields of applied linguistics (Schubert, 2016). A 'narrow' view of register is one where vocabulary alone is seen as the defining characteristic across different registers:

> Linguistic varieties that are linked [...] to particular occupations or topics can be termed registers [...] Registers are usually characterised entirely, or almost so, by vocabulary differences. (Trudgill, 2000: p. 81)

This narrow view of register variation as simple "vocabulary differences" does not however consider the lexico-grammatical, social or functional contexts in which the language of a register is produced. Instead, a wider perspective on register is required that takes these factors into account, involving a description of a given text's situational features, linguistic features, and how mappings of form and function constitute the conventional associations that typify that register. This is exemplified in Figure 1.1 from Biber (1994).

FUNCTIONS

SITUATIONAL FEATURES ⟷ AND ⟷ LINGUISTIC FORMS

CONVENTIONS

Figure 1.1 Components of register studies (Biber, 1994: p. 32)

1.2.2 Analysing register

The 'wide' view of register described in the previous section has been investigated through the lens of three main methodological approaches within the field of register studies. Those working under the umbrella of Systemic Functional Linguistics

(SFL) analyse texts and language features for the purpose of labelling their functions according to the *field* (subject matter), *mode* (medium of transmission) and *tenor* (relationship between participants and context) in which they are produced. This generally involves manually labelling individual or groups of linguistic features found within texts along increasingly complex functional taxonomies (e.g. the appraisal framework, Martin & White, 2003). Critics of this approach see the kind of open-ended parameters that constitute many SFL-based taxonomies as being imprecise, as the number of possible values for each parameter may be infinite according to the subjectivity of the coder or complexity of the function. This can make it difficult to offer a reliable characterisation of an individual register across different researchers or to meaningfully compare one register with that of another in certain cases.

To more objectively account for register variation, one has to be able to precisely quantify the distribution of assigned classes of linguistic features, and reveal how their "representative selection" serves functional or conventional purposes (Biber, 1994: p. 35). This goal has been primarily addressed in the literature through a corpus-based Multidimensional Analysis approach (MDA, Biber, 1988, 1995, 2006a; Biber & Conrad, 2009). As a methodology, MDA involves the use of automated natural language processing techniques including syntactic parsing, part-of-speech tagging and the annotation of functional lexico-grammatical features such as hedges or stance markers on large representative language corpora to derive the co-occurrence of lexico-grammatical features which serve particular functions (or 'dimensions'). Because these features are discrete and countable, their relative co-occurrence is both readily quantifiable and easily comparable across other text types and registers. The MDA approach has been used to determine the characteristics of a range of general registers (Biber, 1988, 1995), academic registers (Biber, 2006a; Biber & Gray, 2010, 2016; Crosthwaite, 2016), registers on the web (Biber & Kurjian, 2007), registers, genres and style (Biber & Conrad, 2009), and historical register variation (Biber & Gray, 2013). This pioneering work has also led to a wealth of related studies using MDA to determine register variation across disciplinary texts (e.g. Nesi, 2009; Nesi & Gardner, 2012; Gardner, Nesi & Biber, 2018; Crossley, Kyle & Römer, 2019).

Another corpus-based approach to the study of academic registers is found in the work of Ken Hyland, who, as you might know from the foreword to this volume, was chair professor for applied linguistics and director of the Centre for Applied English Studies (CAES) at the University of Hong Kong – the context of the present study – during the creation of our ESAP curriculum. Hyland's contribution to the corpus-based research of academic registers focuses on how academic writers organise their texts while dialogically engaging with their target readership, with both achieved through the use of *metadiscourse* (Hyland, 2005; Hyland & Tse,

2004). While a number of metadiscourse features are also present in MDA analyses (e.g. hedges), writing under a metadiscourse framework is seen more as a form of social engagement, with studies on academic writing in particular "revealing the ways that writers project themselves into their discourse to signal their attitude towards both the propositional content and the audience of the text" (Hyland & Tse, 2004: p. 156). Hyland's work has revealed how a discipline may in fact be characterised by the linguistic and rhetorical choices made within its literature (Hyland, 1998, 2004a, 2008), how these choices may be changing over time (Hyland & Jiang, 2016a, 2016b), as well as how novice and second language writers struggle to reproduce these choices due to linguistic deficits and a lack of awareness of academic and disciplinary conventions (e.g. Hyland, 2004b, 2007, 2012). Hyland's influence has also extended to our own work on the language features responsible for interaction and organisation in disciplinary academic registers (Crosthwaite, Cheung & Jiang, 2017; Crosthwaite & Jiang, 2017).

In terms of our personal methodological approach, the work in this volume takes cues from Biber's MDA analyses, Hyland's metadiscourse model, and the incorporation of newer computational approaches to the analysis of texts within the dentistry register. Evert (2018), in a recent lecture at the University of Birmingham, stated that much research in corpus linguistics still relies on 50-year-old techniques, including Sinclairian collocation and keyword analyses, combined with manual interpretation of concordance output. MDA approaches to register variation are still largely the same as they were in Biber (1988), with many analyses still using Biber's (1988) dimensions as a source of comparison (although we also adopt these at one point in this volume). Since the 1990s, advances in computational processing power, the internet, natural language processing (NLP) technology and the fantastic work of corpus linguists in developing tools to analyse available corpora have led to a revolution in the study and analysis of register across disciplines. More recently, developments in data visualization and automated NLP-driven analyses are providing exciting new perspectives on language that, while often quite removed from the actual object of study, can in fact actually help us better understand registers and genres in fresh and unexpected ways. This is part of a technique known as 'distant reading' (Moretti, 2013). While our volume includes more traditional forms of register analysis in Chapters 2 and 3, it is also our intention to showcase new innovations in corpus analysis from a relatively left-field perspective, shedding new light on patterns and trends within dentistry writing that might have hitherto remained undiscovered (e.g. the final analysis of Chapter 3, and the entirety of Chapter 4).

We need to clearly state at the outset that the present volume does not fall under the umbrella of the research areas known as 'health text mining' or 'medical informatics', which involve the use of NLP tools to automatically analyse electronic patient records for diagnoses, medication histories, laboratory test results or radiological imaging data. Such data is typically processed to augment clinical decision-making, including drug interactions, standards development, clinical outcomes, genetic variation and a myriad of other practical applications (e.g. Jensen, Jensen & Brunak, 2012; Cohen & Hersch, 2005). The field shares much in common with register studies given it is driven by the use of NLP tools on language data including entity recognition, POS tagging, tokenisation, and machine learning applications that can use the mined data to predict clinical outcomes.

However, our work in this volume differs from that of medical data mining in a number of respects. The main difference is that medical data mining typically deals with unstructured data (Feldman & Sanger, 2007), while the corpus data used in this volume have been carefully selected in order to be maximally representative of the genres we have chosen for analysis. Additionally, due to the legal and ethical considerations involved with accessing patient record data (or even undergraduate's novice attempts at writing case reports, for example), our volume focuses on professional academic writing within the dentistry discipline, as well as the submissions our dentistry undergraduate students provided for their ESAP course assessments. There is a great deal of writing done by dentists in practicing clinics that would be of interest to ESAP professionals for teaching purposes, including summaries of laboratory test results, or patient record histories. However, privacy and ethical concerns limit the genres and data we can access for corpus analysis to data that is already in the public domain and written for the academy. It also goes without saying that while we hope our volume helps novice dentists to be successful writers for their discipline, we would be very surprised if our findings actually improved clinical practice!

One other caveat to our approach in terms of the corpus-based research undertaken in the first section of this volume is that all corpus tools and applications used should be freely available, and not require any extensive programming knowledge to use. One of the great things about being a corpus linguist today is the great wealth of available corpora and open-source software already developed by and for the research community. This applies both to available corpora as well as to corpus query tools, taggers, builders, annotators, visualisers and analysers, with the entire suite growing daily. While programming abilities can help corpus researchers to "allow the posing of corpus-based research questions never asked before" (Cortes & Csomay, 2015: p. xv), so many good tools and resources are now available that corpus-based research can be both conducted and replicated even by relative newcomers to the field, including ESAP/EGAP professionals seeking to conduct similar analyses of their own target disciplinary discourses. The tools and other software are all fully cited where appropriate throughout the volume, with URLs provided as footnotes for others to trial these tools themselves.

1.2.3 Genres for analysis

Given the conceptual, empirical and methodological basis for the study of the register of dentistry writing described in the previous section, in order to proceed further we must address the possible range of recurrent disciplinary text types, or *genres*, suitable for analysis within the dentistry discipline. There has been much disagreement in the literature about the complimentary/opposing nature of genres and registers, and we do not have space in this chapter to discuss this disagreement further (we refer the reader to Biber & Conrad, 2009, for a detailed discussion of this topic). In this volume, we follow the definition of Dorgeloh and Wanner (2010) in that a genre is a type of social action used for individual tasks within a register, and the frequency and distribution of the linguistic features of a genre constitute a kind of "patterned practice" that shapes the overall register. Dorgeloh (2016: p. 43) further argues that a genre analysis "logically subsumes and pre-determines a register analysis" in that there is a hybridity of features typical of more general registers (e.g. narrative features) within specific genres. Rather, it is the function of specific genres (or "social event", *ibid.*) that can account for how a specific register (e.g. the 'language of dentistry') may be realised. Continuing the musical analogy from Section 1.2.1, Schubert (2016) likens genre to "the specific musical piece chosen by the church organist", while register is the "music" itself (p. 5).

In selecting the genres to be analysed in this volume, a primary consideration is that of the author's "voices", or different linguistic means through which the author represents themselves and the social event they are engaged in (Mishler, 1984; Dorgeloh, 2016: p. 43). Working on the medical register, Dorgeloh compared corpora of 'illness blogs', case reports and a type of open discussion forum article found within the *Journal of the American Medical Association*. Dorgeloh found that while narrative features cut across each of these three genres, it is variation in the use and frequency of these features that is representative of the 'voice' (e.g. 'doctor', 'medicine', 'patient') utilised by the writer at specific points across the genres analysed. Schryer, Lingard and Spafford (2007: p. 22) in their investigation of oral medical case presentations suggest that in the acquisition of disciplinary genres, one is acquiring both the "regulated" resources of their profession as well as "regularised" ways of knowing. Both types of resources play a key role in the formation of professional identity, with "regulated" resources externally controlled, while "regularised" resources represent more of a discipline-internal, socialised set of behaviours and "voices".

The genres selected for analysis should therefore encompass a variety of the "voices" a practicing dentist might employ while writing within the discipline, whether writing as a dentist, as a researcher, as a provider of a visible and essential community service, or as an undergraduate student. To achieve this, we selected three genres for analysis that undergraduates would be expected to frequently encounter during their studies and be expected to be engaged in writing shortly upon graduation, and that constitutes a unique "voice" through which the students can realise their new identities as members of their discipline. These were the experimental research paper, novice and professional research reports within the domain of Dental Public Health, and the case report. Chapters 2 and 3 deal with register analysis at a broader level, involving MDA analyses (Chapters 2 and 3) as well as analysis of metadiscoursal features (Chapter 3), while Chapter 4 narrows the focus of analysis to explore disciplinary vs. non-disciplinary senses of lexis within the case report genre via automated NLP-based processes. We now describe the rationale for each chapter in Section 1 in turn.

1.3 Chapter 2 – 'Extracting' the linguistic dimensions of dentistry experimental research articles

Dentistry is a sub-category of the physical and life science domains. The goal of scientific research writing is to communicate new findings and discoveries to researchers in the discipline, and the key genre used for this communication is that of the experimental research article. For dentistry, experimental research papers can include new procedures, new materials, new medicines, and new ways of solving existing problems, with the author's 'voice' ranging from that of 'practicing dentist', 'empirical researcher', 'educator', and 'colleague'. However, Biber and Gray (2016) suggest that this very process of discovery is one of the main causes of difficulty for novice readers of academic science writing, which is laden with technical vocabulary and written so as to maximally compress complex information into very short spans of text. While experts in the field are used to deciphering technical language and unpacking this compressed information as trained readers, novices to academic science writing face a daunting task made even more difficult in contexts where such writing is to be read and understood by second language users of the target language.

As one of the most frequently occurring genres of academic writing, corpus-based analyses of academic research papers have focused on a wide range of linguistic features, including the derivation of academic wordlists (e.g. Coxhead, 2000; Coxhead & Nation, 2001), phraseological patterns or lexical bundles (Cortes, 2004, Hyland, 2008), and student writing (e.g. Gardner & Nesi, 2012; Hardy & Römer, 2013), and have done so using a variety of methodological frameworks. In terms of MDA studies on the register of research articles, Gray (2015) utilised corpora to compare research articles across six different disciplines, finding significant cross-disciplinary variation in elaborative and compressive structures alongside lexico-grammatical variation of forms including *if*-conditional clauses and linking adverbials. Biber and Gray (2016) found significant variation in the use of noun participles functioning as pre-modifiers (e.g. *ribosome-binding* activities) across the popular science, social science and specialist science sub-registers of science writing, with heavy use of this form in the specialist sub-register. Specific to medical research articles, which are an influential and prolific source of academic writing generally (Gotti & Salager-Meyer, 2006), Biber and Finegan (1994) explored the use of *that*-verb complements, modals, pronouns and tense before employing an MDA analysis comparing medical research writing to that of other registers. Non-MDA studies on medical research articles have focused on rhetorical functions of lexis within Hyland's metadiscourse approach, including analyses of hedging (Dahl, 2004), and engagement markers (Herrando-Rodrigo, 2010), while others have adopted SFL-based approaches including Martin and White's (2003) appraisal framework (Fryer, 2013).

While it is possible that some of the above studies have included research articles from the dentistry discipline within their data, there is a lack of corpus-based research that has looked at specifically at experimental research articles in dentistry. Kostenko (2016) claims that different medical subdisciplines hold their own values, beliefs, attitudes, customs and behavioural patterns which have "lead to even further immersion of learners into the knowledge and culture of their own professional group" (p. 238), yet, despite this, dentistry is still a critically underexplored discipline among studies of other medical registers. Carlson (2000) is a major exception, analysing a corpus of 1,400 dentistry research abstracts for word frequency and collocation patterns, with Carlson specifically calling for the results to feature into ESAP materials for L2 dentistry writers. In addition, Basturkmen (2012) focused on rhetorical move structure within the discussion section of dentistry research articles as compared with articles from applied linguistics. Basturkmen notes a similar move structure between the two disciplines, yet more importance is placed on evaluating rather than explaining results in the dentistry discussion sections. Despite these interesting findings, Baskturkmen (2012: p. 135) notes "very little appears to be known in applied linguistics about research writing in dentistry [and] published information about research writing written by dentists also appears to be rare". Moreover, both Carlson (2000) and Baskturkmen (2012) have only analysed specific subsections of dentistry research articles rather than full texts in their respective research.

Chapter 2 of this volume therefore presents what is likely the first large-scale corpus-based analysis of full experimental dentistry research articles, with an equivalent reference corpus of research articles taken from general medical journals for comparison. We adopt an MDA approach to determine the functional grouping of linguistic features of dentistry research articles against those of Biber's

(1988) dimensions, as well as conduct a new MDA that determines a set of dimensions specific to dentistry research articles. We also reveal the keywords and phraseological features specific to dentistry research articles as compared with those from general medical journals, which form a teachable list of such items for ESAP purposes.

1.4 Chapter 3 – Persuasive stories?: Professional and novice research reports for Dental Public Health

The dentistry discipline plays a highly visible role in the maintenance of public health within the local community where dentists practice. While studies on academic registers have focused extensively on research papers, one lesser-explored area for analysis is where the research focuses on the interactions of that discipline with the general public, or where such research is charged with collecting the opinions of the general public on practices within that discipline (Crawford, Adami, Johnson, Knight, Knoernschild, Obrez, Patson, Punwani, Zaki, & Licari, 2007). As most research papers written for dentistry are seemingly impenetrable for the general public – if one were to pick up a research paper on chemical reactions to certain tooth implants, for example – reporting on the findings of interactions between the community and the discipline it serves can be considered an essential social event for the discipline, a form of "knowledge exchange" (Mitton, Adair, McKenzie, Patten & Waye Perry, 2007: p. 729). Within dentistry, this area of research writing is termed Dental Public Health (DPH), which unlike the majority of dentistry research writing, deals with non-clinical issues surrounding the prevention of oral disease alongside issues relating to community beliefs and practice regarding general dental health. The goal of the writer in this area is not simply to report on these interactions as one would expect in a clinical research paper, but to use the findings of the research to "advocate for public health policy, legislation, and regulations to protect and promote the public's oral health, and overall health" (Altman & Mascarenhas, 2016: p. s18). The goal of this specialisation within dentistry research writing in particular is that of "aligning the goals of the patient and the physician" (Winker, 2006: p. 2888), with a view to eventually disseminating the findings via the media to the general public, informing them of potential dangers to their health, reducing risks and instructing them to live healthier lifestyles (McGuire, 1984: p. 311). As such, those trained in Dental Public Health must also "be proficient in communication to interact effectively with multiple audiences" (Hernandez, Rosenstock & Gebbie, 2003: p. 8). The 'voices' employed this genre are not only those of the 'practitioner' and 'researcher', but also those of 'reporter' and 'advocate' for the promotion of DPH on behalf of the dentistry discipline.

Such is the importance of DPH within the discipline as a whole that an increasingly large proportion of dental schools globally now incorporate community-based experiential learning opportunities in DPH for their students (Crawford et al., 2007). This is also the case in the context of the present volume, with the University of Hong Kong offering this opportunity in the fifth and final year of undergraduate dental studies in the form of an experiential learning DPH capstone project titled the *Community Dental Health Project* (CHP), which has been in place as an assessment in the undergraduate program since 1984.

However, in many L2 contexts there is no accompanying ESAP provision for this purpose (Morse & Nakahara, 2001), a consideration that lead to the redevelopment of the ESAP course featured in the present volume. The new course focuses primarily on teaching the linguistic features and rhetorical functions for this CHP , as part of the *English-in-the-discipline* (ED) suite of ESAP courses that spanned numerous faculties across the university (Hyland, 2014, see also the foreword and Chapter 5 of this volume). Preparing students to undertake the CHP assessment is a considerable challenge for the ESAP professional, given that the research paper summarising the CHP must be written entirely in English by a cohort with no experience of writing DPH research articles, and for whom very few who hold English as a mother tongue, and with Cantonese as the primary language of communication between the novice researchers and the Hong Kong community they are to interact with and report on for the CHP.

Chapter 3 of this volume therefore reports on three analyses involving data taken from Dental Public Health-focused research, with a view to characterizing the rhetorical patterns of language use employed by both novice and professional writers. The first such analysis involves an MDA of a corpus of professionally-written Dental Public Health research papers drawn from the journal *Community Dental Health,* which is a key international journal publishing on a wide spectrum of public health issues in dentistry that are highly relevant to the CHPs. The MDA of this data located five dimensions of groupings of rhetorical features (to be revealed in the chapter), which were then used for comparison with a corpus of completed CHP assessments taken from our novice dental undergraduates.

Our second analysis of this data involves the derivation of three specific lexical features involved in the presentation of the author's stance (Hyland, 2005; Biber, 2006b) across both professional and novice corpora; namely hedges, boosters and self-mention. Hedges allow writers to express their lack of commitment to the certainty of the information given (e.g. 'this data *may* help to …'), while boosters allow writers to express their confidence about the validity of a proposition (e.g. 'this data *proves* that …') (Holmes, 1988; Hu & Cao, 2015; Hyland, 2005). Hedges and boosters are a central rhetorical device in science discourse, used to gain communal adherence to knowledge claims and build interpersonal solidarity with readers (Hyland, 1999), and there have been numerous studies on how novice and L2 writers handle these features in academic writing (Lancaster, 2016; Crosthwaite, Cheung & Jiang, 2017).

The final analysis of the CHP data in this chapter involves the use of an alternative, automated approach to rhetorical analysis. Here, we utilise the freely available *Ubiqu+Ity*[2] , which is an online text analysis environment for corpus-based rhetorical analysis made available through the University of Wisconsin-Madison. This web-based software annotates text files for features present under the *Docuscope* dictionary (Kaufer, Ishizaki, Butler & Collins 2004; Kaufer, Geisler, Vlachos & Ishizaki, 2006), comprised of "over 40 million" (n.d.)[3] linguistic patterns of English classified into over 100 categories of rhetorical effects including 'narrative', 'citation' and 'description'. Together, the three analyses provided in this chapter seek to characterise the rhetorical functions employed by both professional and novice writers in detailing their interactions with local communities, and the way their advocacy for Dental Public Health issues within that community is disseminated in written form.

1.5 Chapter 4 – Understanding disciplinary vs. non-disciplinary terminology: Insights from the dentistry case report genre

Case reports describe, in detail, actual clinical procedures that take place in dental surgeries. They are used to outline information about patients' conditions, the decision-making processes that influenced dentists' choice of procedures, the materials used for procedures, the procedures themselves, the immediate results of these procedures, and any directions and guidelines for future follow-up procedures. These reports are typically used by healthcare professionals "to communicate the salient details of patient cases to one another" (Schryer, Lingard, Spafford & Garwood, 2003: p. 63), while Kostenko (2017) suggests case reports "promote social networking among dentists and dental communities [and] serve as a stepping stone for further trials and research" (p. 1). Case reports have an additional function of "stating verifiable events" (Dorgeloh, 2016: p. 52), acting as written evidence of procedure that can be called upon in case of procedural error or investigation of malpractice.

There have already been a number of corpus-based studies of medical case reports. Salager-Meyer (1991) compared a corpus of medical case reports with

2. version 1.2, https://vep.cs.wisc.edu/ubiq/

3. https://www.cmu.edu/dietrich/english/research/docuscope.html

corpora of research papers, editorials and reviews, considering case reports and research papers as similar in terms of the frequency of hedging devices present as compared with editorials and reviews. In later work, Salager-Meyer (1994) analysed a corpus of 15 case report articles to determine the use of hedges by section of the reports (e.g. introduction, results, discussion), finding variation in the type and frequency of hedging devices used by section across case reports and research articles. Dorgeloh (2016) included medical case reports in her analysis of the medical register, noting that this genre often employs the patient rather than the doctor as the clausal topic under discussion. This leads to two additional 'voices' writers employ within this genre, namely the voice of 'medicine' regarding the doctor's "translation" of patients' complaints (Hurwitz, 2006: p. 216), and the voice of 'disease', regarding the complaint itself, for example:

> A 27-year old Hispanic woman presented [...] with a sudden onset of shortness of breath and increased difficulty in moving her right arm [...] She also complained of chest pains that we localised behind the sternum. (Dorgeloh, 2016: p. 53)

Despite being a crucial genre within the medical and dental disciplines, mastering these different voices can be a difficult task for students of dentistry. Schryer et al. (2003) suggest that due to conflicting roles of agency for medical students as both 'student' and 'doctor', student adoption of the rhetorical and linguistic choices required for case reports can lead to medical students "learning to classify in quite specific ways, behaviours that could negatively affect communication with their patients" (p. 62). This occurs, for example, if they are misunderstanding complex terminology present in case reports and using such terminology in discussion with patients, or relaying information to patients using the same rhetorical structures reserved for professional case reports. Lingard, Garwood, Schryer and Spafford (2003), in their study on features of uncertainty across professional and student presentations of case reports, note differences between professional and novice rhetorical features of uncertainty within such reports. Uncertainty in professional presentations originated mainly from limits of evidence, patient's accounts, professional agreement, and scientific knowledge, while student accounts of uncertainty tended to focus on a lack of personal knowledge. In a qualitative study on the perceptions of Ukrainian dentistry students on academic writing, Kostenko (2018) claims that writing for genres other than research articles (including case reports) can be associated with language anxiety as students leave their relative comfort zones when grappling with a new set of organisational and rhetorical practices. In fact, the effects of poor use of disciplinary language features leads many case report submissions to be routinely rejected from high impact journals in the field such as *Journal of Conservative Dentistry* (Gopikrishna, 2010).

Other than Kostenko's (2017) doctoral thesis (analysing a corpus of just 20 dentistry case reports), there are no other corpus-based studies that have tackled case reports specifically within the dentistry discipline. However, it is here that our analysis of case reports departs from those of previous research in terms of both the linguistic focus as well as methodology. Rather than working manually with smaller corpora, we present three automated analyses of a large corpus of over 800 dentistry case report articles taken from the online open-access journal *Case Reports in Dentistry,* spanning over 1,300,000 words. As the structural and register features of case reports have been documented in previous research (e.g. Dorgeloh 2016), and following on from the concerns raised by Schryer et al. (2003) and Lingard, Garwood, Schryer and Spafford (2003) about difficulties for novice dentists in dealing with disciplinary lexis, our intention in this chapter is primarily focus on disciplinary lexical features. Our approach here is rather left-field and experimental in corpus studies of academic writing, in that our analyses start from a corpus-driven, rather than corpus-based perspective, letting the data guide the scope of our analysis with few preconceived notions of what we expect to find.

The first analysis of the data in this chapter involves a *sentiment analysis*, using the *SEANCE: Sentiment Analysis and Cognition Engine* (Crossley, Kyle & McNamara, 2017). A sentiment analysis involves the use of natural language processing procedures in determining the attitude, polarity and emotional content of the target text. We compared the features derived using *SEANCE* from the case report corpus against those of the dental research article corpus we present in Chapter 2, with the results of this analysis suggesting that case reports are significantly more likely to contain negative adjectives, positive nouns and verbs, and sentiments related to 'well-being', and, surprisingly, 'fear and disgust'. This approach allows the researcher to determine the range of non-disciplinary attitudes and emotions inherent within disciplinary lexis. This knowledge is important for novice professionals as noted in Schryer et al. (2003) in terms of the clash between 'student' and 'doctor' linguistic identities adopted during clinical training. This knowledge is ever more important for L2 users, who are likely to have acquired the non-disciplinary sentiment of disciplinary lexis prior to understanding disciplinary usage, which may make the initial task of reading and writing case reports more difficult than it would be under an L1-only condition. Our goal here is avoid the potential for 'patient' and 'doctor' misalignment in terms of the attitude, emotion and import of disciplinary terminology as it used in case reports and as it may be used in communication with real patients during clinical practice.

The second analysis of this chapter involves the use of a semantic tagger (the *UCREL Semantic Analysis System*, USAS, Rayson, Archer, Piao & McEnery, 2004) within the online corpus analysis portal *Wmatrix* (Rayson, 2008). This software automatically analyses the semantic information of a corpus according to 21 semantic domains or "discourse fields" (*ibid*). These domains include those that may be understood as more central to medical science writing, such as 'the body and the individual' and 'substances, materials, objects and equipment', as well as domains one might not automatically associate with the medical register such as 'movement, location, travel and transport', 'numbers and measurement', 'time' and 'psychological states, actions and processes'. Again, knowing the disciplinary vs. non-disciplinary senses of terminology embedded within case report writing could be very important for novice professionals – especially L2 professionals – to understand, both in terms of their writing of the case report and in terms of their interactions with patients during clinical practice. In very recent research, Whiteside and Wharton (2019: p. 1) also suggest that from a practitioner perspective, a corpus-based semantic approach "uncovers meaning-focused lexico-grammatical features of very high value due to their extremely regular occurrence within student texts". The frequency of annotated semantic categories and items from the case report corpus is then compared with those of a 1,000,000 corpus of general written English (the *BNC Written Sampler*, 1999) so as to determine the key semantic subdomains associated with case report writing as compared with general written English, and any specific keywords arising from these semantic domains.

The final analysis of this data compares the keywords of the case report corpus against those derived from the corpus of dentistry research articles that was outlined in Chapter 2, using the keyword visualisation software *Scattertext* (Kessler, 2017). The triangulation of these three automated analyses provides insights into the case report writing genre that would likely have remained undiscovered through more traditional analyses, resulting in a left-field but teachable set of keywords, sentiments and semantic domains that can be used to train novice writers to understand disciplinary and non-disciplinary senses of the language of case reports.

1.6 Introduction to Section 2

The second section of the volume deals with how the data from Section 1 was used to drive innovations in ESAP materials and pedagogy, and how undergraduate students of dentistry themselves analysed the data for the purposes of writing for the discipline. This was achieved both indirectly through corpus-derived updates and additions to course content and curricula, and directly (Leech, 1997) through hands-on corpus use by ESAP students in the form of "data-driven learning" (DDL, Johns, 1991). Chapter 5 deals with the rationale for and implementation of a new purpose-built corpus platform and associated DDL activities into the ESAP dentistry disciplinary writing programme, while Chapter 6 deals with the actual usage and evaluation of students' corpus use for DDL. The concluding Chapter 7 reports on the perceptions of students, ESAP tutors and disciplinary content tutors on these corpus-based applications, before describing our outlook for future research.

1.7 Chapter 5 – Data-driven dentistry: Corpora, ESAP, and writing-to-learn

Chapter 5 of this volume details how corpora were implemented into ESAP as part of 'writing-to-learn' for the discipline (Manchón, 2011). This ESAP provision is currently realised at the University of Hong Kong (HKU) through the introduction of *English in the Discipline* (ED) disciplinary writing courses spanning nine faculties (Hyland, 2014). ED promotes the enhancement of undergraduates' academic literacy skills that can be applied and transferred to target disciplinary fields. This innovation was necessitated by changes in Hong Kong's education system from a 3-year to 4-year undergraduate degree program (5 years for dentistry) resulting in one year less of secondary education, as well as a shift to Cantonese or Mandarin as the medium-of-instruction in most Hong Kong secondary schools since the 1997 handover of sovereignty from the UK to China. This is despite professionals spending much of their time reading and writing for the discipline in English (Evans, 2011).

Previous ESAP provision prior to ED focused on demonstrating skills in oral and written English. This was very much in the 'learning-to-write' mode, with activities based on a variety of communication skills featured in dentistry-related real-life scenarios, but that was primarily focused on local rather than global issues with student writing, lacked opportunities for meaningful engagement with written content, and was organised largely externally to – rather than in parallel with – disciplinary content provision and assessments. The shift to ED was that of a shift to 'writing-to-learn', with a new focus on getting students to become acquainted with disciplinary language features and discourse practices in order to "take on new roles and engage with knowledge in new ways" (Hyland, 2014: p. 142) as they learn about the discipline through specially selected writing activities designed to reflect discipline-specific social practices and epistemologies, conducted in tandem with the disciplinary capstone assessment. From the outset, ED courses required effective collaboration between the ESAP teachers and content teachers from faculties, ideally so that the learning activities in the ESAP could be contextualised through concurrent activities in the disciplinary content courses. This was the case for the dentistry ED course, where ESAP and disciplinary supervisors worked together on different elements of the Community Health Project (CHP) capstone, the former dealing with writing the CHP report, and the latter concerned with the research topic and organising the research project as a whole.

Corpora have a significant role to play in ED provision by exposing students to empirical evidence about language that allows them to understand the characteristic language features involved in producing disciplinary genres of writing, thus enhancing their understanding of the complexities of literacy within their target disciplinary field. While the development of ESAP materials without corpora tend to rely on a course developer's intuitive sense of what students need to learn (at least, without significant input from disciplinary tutors), corpora can provide educators with numerous authentic examples of target disciplinary language. The corpora may then themselves be used by students to discover the key features of disciplinary language in use. However, the initial implementation of a corpus component during the first iteration of the dentistry ED course received criticism due to a slow corpus query platform and limited corpus functionality, where concordances were the sole form of access to the corpus data.

To resolve these issues, a redesign of the dentistry ESAP course involved the creation of a new, multifunctional and highly visual corpus query platform, alongside a suite of carefully sequenced in-class and supplemental ESAP activities. The target language items were based in part on the findings from our corpus analyses of research articles (Chapter 2) and the findings from our comparison of the professional and learner corpora of Dental Public Health articles (Chapter 3), as well as our study on disciplinary lexis within case reports (Chapter 4). This information was used to shape activities that required students to directly query our disciplinary corpora themselves as part of a data-driven learning pedagogical approach (DDL, Johns, 1991).

DDL is now increasingly used to enhance the teaching of EAP (e.g. Crosthwaite, 2017; Chen & Flowerdew, 2018; Cotos, 2014; Lee & Swales, 2006; Tono, Satake & Muira, 2014, Yoon & Hirvela, 2004), and is generally experienced in the form of structured tasks requiring the consultation of corpus data with the aim of 'noticing' (Schmidt, 1990) the statistical patterns of contextualised language in use, including data on word frequency, collocation and keyness. DDL has been lauded as an approach rich in opportunity for focus on form (Long, 1991), in that meaning-focused language learning tasks involving corpus consultation are said to help draw learners' attention to target language features. Combining language output with a range of statistical (and increasingly visual) corpus output is also claimed to resonate with constructivist/connectionist approaches to language learning. One such example is that of chunking (Millar, 2011), where data on collocates and multi-word units are clearly presented in lists, visual charts, heat maps, etc., each of which can facilitate learning. Researchers have also praised DDL as an increasingly relevant pedagogy for modern digitally-oriented learners (Kilgarriff & Grefenstette, 2003; Boulton, 2015), and students' self-guided engagement with corpora during DDL has been shown to improve learner autonomy for resolving language-related problems

(Leńko-Szymańska & Boulton, 2015). Recent meta-analyses of the effectiveness of DDL for language learning (Cobb & Boulton, 2015; Boulton & Cobb, 2017; Lee, Warschauer & Lee, 2018) have found medium to large effect sizes across hundreds of DDL studies and thousands of research participants.

There have already been book-length treatments of DDL for ESAP, even within the *Studies in Corpus Linguistics* series (Gavioli, 2005). Gavioli's work suggests hands-on use of corpora is well-suited for the discovery of disciplinary language features and the promotion of learner autonomy for language learning. Her work describes the "search and discovery" (p. 2) experiences of corpus exploration by ESAP undergraduate students of advanced L2 proficiency, while describing for the reader the kind of tasks that allow for this exploration to occur. Gavioli compiled specialised corpora of medical research articles including subcorpora on specific conditions (e.g. Hepatitis C, Gastric Cancer), spanning approximately 250,000 words in total, with a view to using this data for DDL. Our volume seeks to build considerably on Gavioli's work in a number of respects, notably in terms of the larger corpora created for this volume, and the incorporation of an improved DDL user interface featuring data visualisation and learner analytics that were simply not available to researchers a decade ago. An edited volume also in the *Studies in Corpus Linguistics* series (Boulton, Carter-Thomas and Rowley-Jolivet, 2012) has dealt with DDL for ESAP in its final three chapters (Williams, 2012, for the sciences; Birch-Beccas & Cooke, 2012, for discourse moves; and Boulton, 2012 with a review of empirical studies), while another recent edited volume on general ESAP research (Flowerdew & Costley, 2017) has also devoted its final three chapters to the use of DDL for ESAP, including Anthony (2017a) using DDL for STEM technical writing, Chun (2017) using DDL for business memo writing, and Lockwood (2017) using corpora for the assessment of disciplinary writing.

Both recognising and building upon the valuable contribution of such research, Chapter 5 describes the introduction of DDL pedagogy into the dentistry ED course across two years of instruction. We document the initial implementation of corpus-based materials into the ED course, what this involved, and describe why it initially failed to meet the expectations of both students and faculty. We then describe why we doubled-down on the direct use of corpora for the ED course despite our initial disappointment, before outlining the functionality of the new purpose-built ED corpus platform (see also Crosthwaite, Wong & Cheung, 2019) and presenting the DDL activities that students completed while 'writing-to-learn' for the discipline.

1.8 Chapter 6 – Putting it into (dental) practice: User engagement with dentistry corpora and DDL

Chapter 6 of this volume reports on findings arising from the usage statistics generated via the purpose-built online corpus query platform outlined in Chapter 5, charting dentistry students' actual engagement with this platform in terms of their corpus query and platform usage habits. Despite a wealth of DDL studies focusing on student or teacher perceptions of DDL, or experimental works detailing improvements in accuracy or lexical knowledge, very little is currently known about students' corpus query habits for disciplinary writing (Hafner & Candlin, 2007), although studies collecting data on actual corpus usage and queries are now finding their way into the literature (Gaskell & Cobb, 2004; Hafner & Candlin, 2007; Yoon, 2008; Pérez-Paredes, Sánchez-Tornel, Alcaraz Calero, and Jiménez, 2011; Crosthwaite, Wong & Cheung, 2019). The majority of DDL studies have used established and popular corpus query interfaces such as *AntConc* (Anthony, 2014), the Brigham-Young University (BYU) suite of online corpora (Davies, 2004), *SketchEngine* (Kilgarriff, Rychly, Smrz, & Tugwell, 2004) or *SketchEngine for Language Learning* (Baisa & Suchomel, 2014), while other studies employ the use of more rudimentary in-house online concordancers (e.g. Hafner & Candlin, 2007). Neither type easily facilitates the collection of data on corpus usage history, nor – more importantly – data of the actual corpus queries made and who made them. Without this data, there is a large gap in what we currently know about what students actually *do* when consulting corpora during DDL. However, our purpose-built DDL system as described in Chapter 5 of this volume (see also Crosthwaite, Wong & Cheung, 2019), allowed us to track and document users' query histories and usage habits, providing a window into the actual process underlying students' engagement with DDL that has hitherto yet to be adequately quantified and documented. Chapter 6, therefore, is devoted to describing this data, in what is a rare attempt to track students' idiosyncratic DDL query histories and platform engagement for disciplinary writing purposes. We describe the frequency and form of queries made using the corpus platform, particularly noting where the students had gone beyond the prescribed course materials to generate queries of their own making. We look at which corpus functions students typically employed when making queries, and which functions they tended not to use. Finally, we track the platform usage habits of the most frequent corpus users among the professional and learner corpus data, revealing and characterising their idiosyncrasies while hypothesising their intended goals in querying the available corpora using our platform. We then discuss the implications of this analysis for future iterations of DDL for dentistry, as well as for the application of DDL and ESAP more generally.

1.9 Chapter 7 – Reflections on practice, future directions

We close this volume in Chapter 7 with a qualitative evaluation of what we have achieved through the previous chapters. This evaluation is primarily supported through the thoughts and opinions of the students themselves, focusing on their quantitative and qualitative opinions derived from end-of-course evaluations and one-on-one interviews. We also focus on the comments of the ESAP and disciplinary tutors involved in the dentistry ED course, providing an outlet for their voices on the value of ESAP for the dentistry profession generally, and, specifically, the contribution that corpora can make to that endeavour. We then proceed to look forward to future directions regarding the role and use of corpora for ESAP in light of advances in new technologies, emerging disciplinary contexts, and synergies with language professionals, as well as consider the changing landscape of EAP provision in an increasingly online world.

SECTION I

The language of dentistry – A corpus-based exploration of language features across the dentistry register

CHAPTER 2

'Extracting' the linguistic dimensions of dentistry experimental research articles

2.1 Introduction

This chapter presents a cross-corpus comparison of experimental research articles written for key journals within the dentistry discipline, compared with those written for a general medical readership. While the experimental research article is a genre common to both dentistry and general medical fields, there may be tacit textual structures and linguistic features that are representative of – or even constitutive of – individual disciplinary fields. Genres such as research articles may be viewed as "places of struggle to establish agency", and uncovering disciplinary differences within the *same* genre may reveal the "constellation of strategies" that disciplinary writers use which are appropriate for the genre as well as appropriate for the discipline (Schryer, Lingard, Spafford & Garwood, 2003: p. 91).

Aside from case reports (Chapter 4), experimental research articles are among the very first professional genres that students of dentistry are exposed to in their disciplinary content courses, and it is likely they will read tens, if not hundreds of such articles during their degree. Internalising the structure and linguistic features of research articles is therefore crucial to students' understanding of much of the disciplinary content they are exposed to at university, as well as their eventual ability to write for and contribute to the discipline. Such is the importance of this task that it constitutes one of the primary learning outcomes of the dentistry English-in-the-discipline course featured in this volume, which requires students to "use appropriate language to present research findings based on extensive and relevant review of literature, research design, data collection, findings, and recommendations" (CAES9350 ED materials, n.d.). In an accompanying introductory video to the course, the Dean of the Faculty of Dentistry is also quoted as saying the course "supports students' knowledge of disciplinary research and expertise in documenting research findings". Both disciplinary tutors and ESAP professionals are acutely aware that understanding – and eventually writing – research articles is an important part of students' disciplinary enculturation, significantly contributing towards the establishment of their identity or "habitus" as professionals (Bazerman, 2002: p. 17).

As mentioned in Chapter 1, Multidimensional Analysis (MDA) takes a 'wide' view of register analysis, in that it allows for the quantifiable characterisation of a range of discrete linguistic features within a corpus. This allows for the register of that corpus to be comprehensively defined on its own terms, and to be effectively characterised through its differences with other registers. As a corpus methodology, MDA involves the use of specialised parsing tools to derive the frequency of an exhaustive array of linguistic features present within a corpus, before exploratory factor analysis (EFA) is used on the output data to observe the statistical co-occurrence of these linguistic features along latent derived factors, or 'dimensions'. These dimensions can be interpreted as performing specific functions characteristic of the register of that corpus, and given their quantifiable nature, readily allow for meaningful cross-corpus and cross-register comparison.

There are two typical methodological variants of MDAs. The first is to compare the linguistic features of a given corpus or set of corpora against a pre-determined set of dimensions as taken from established benchmarks, such as the dimensions or text-types found in Biber (1988, 1989). The second method is to derive a new set of dimensions from a specific corpus (in this case, our corpus of experimental dentistry research articles), and to compare this data with equivalent data from another corpus. This chapter categorises the linguistic features of experimental dentistry research articles using both these approaches. We also employ a variety of other corpus tools to isolate and identify the actual wordings and keywords of the various linguistic categories involved in the MDA analyses within the corpus of dentistry research articles, at the single and multi-word levels.

We have to say at the outset that due to their complex nature, the reporting of MDAs in terms of their methodology and statistical procedures can often be overwhelming for readers who may be unfamiliar with conducting such analyses. While we have provided details on the corpora used in this chapter, the details of the factor analyses conducted for the MDA, as well as the analytical tools used, we do not provide an extensive tutorial in how to conduct an MDA.We would therefore refer the reader to Friginal and Hardy's (2014) extensive guide to conducting MDA in the SPSS statistical package, or Brezina's (2018) *Statistics in Corpus Linguistics: A Practical Guide* which are both excellent resources.

2.2 Corpus construction

Regarding the selection of journals for inclusion into the dentistry and general medical corpora, as an initial step, we simply searched Google using the search terms 'top journals in dentistry' and 'top medical journals' respectively. Browsing these results, an additional consideration was that we needed relatively easy access to PDF versions of the articles in question, preferably via open-access publishing or at least being readily accessible via our institutional credentials. This gave us a list of around 25 journals for each discipline, from which we asked disciplinary tutors to select 10 journals with the best reputation in their field, and that would also be representative of recent trends in disciplinary writing.

Following the selection of journals for analysis, we used citation counts and date of publication as two additional selection criteria for inclusion of individual articles. Given that citation counts are usually inversely correlated with date of publication, we selected a cut-off date that would allow for a certain number of citations to be produced while still selecting 'recent' articles representative of current practice in research report writing. We initially settled on a minimum of 100 citations since the year 2000, and achieving this goal was straightforward when selecting articles within the general medical field, with the final number of citations across the 100 papers selected for that corpus averaging at 1,820 citations since 2000 (with certain papers achieving more than 10,000 citations individually in that time). However, for dentistry – a more specific, narrower discipline – it was harder to maintain this citation/date ratio. Articles from the *Journal of Dental Bioinformatics, Journal of Canadian Dental Health Association, International Journal of Paediatric Dentistry,* and *Acta Odontologica Scandinavica* were often under 100 citations for papers published since 2000. However, the trade-off in citations allowed for the selection of articles from these journals to be more representative of very recent writing, with many papers included in the corpus being published in the last five years. For example, our selection of papers from the *British Dental Journal* were mostly taken from papers published between 2016 and 2017.

In both dentistry and general medical journals, experimental research papers cover real surgical procedures, clinical interventions, clinical trials, testing of statistical models, and testing of new materials, and a broad selection of each type was included in the corpus. As articles in the selected journals can take a wide variety of forms including editorials, position papers or 'news report' type articles for general public dissemination (*Nature,* for example, has numerous articles of this type), we carefully checked each article to ensure it was in fact an experimental research paper. A criterion for inclusion was that the study in question should follow (as much as possible) an AIMRD format (Abstract, Introduction, Method, Results, Discussion). While often very highly cited, meta-analyses of experimental research were often not in the AIMRD format and so were excluded from analysis.

To build the corpus, the freely available *Antfileconverter* (version 1.2.1, Anthony, 2017b)[4] was used to convert the PDF files into plain text file format. With the

4. http://www.laurenceanthony.net/software.html

assistance of a research assistant, these files were then manually stripped of their boilerplates, references and appendices. Only running text was left in the final files, with all figures, diagrams and tables removed from the data. The freely available *Notepad++*[5] was used for this cleaning procedure. This software also helps to easily remove odd characters left in the data as a result of issues with the conversion from PDF format, and which may cause problems for corpus software. The text was then neatly organised into sections to aid analysis, marked up with '##xx' (e.g. ##INTRODUCTION) in the file, with tags following the AIMRD format as closely as possible.

2.3 MDA Version 1: Comparison with Biber's (1988) dimensions

Once the data was cleaned and in the correct format, we used the freely available *Multidimensional Analysis Tagger* (MAT, Version 1.3, Nini, 2015a)[6] to tag and analyse the data. This software is based on the powerful (and accurate) *Stanford Tagger* (Toutanova, Klein, Manning & Singer, 2003), and in the author's words on the MAT website, "replicates Biber's (1988) *Variation across Speech and Writing* tagger for the multidimensional functional analysis of English texts" (n.d.). Running in the Java environment, the software first segments and annotates the data for part-of-speech, then generates a file with a normalised frequency (*n* per 100 tokens) for over 60 linguistic variables found in the corpus. The software then generates standardised z-scores for these variables, before comparing these statistics along five 'dimensions' of linguistic variation sourced from Biber (1988). These dimensions ('involved vs. informational discourse', 'narrative vs. non-narrative concerns', 'explicit vs. situation dependent reference', 'overt expression of persuasion' and 'abstract vs. non-abstract information') act as continua along which certain linguistic features of a given text or corpus may lie, and the relative position of the corpus texts along these continua is taken to be characteristic of their register. MAT produces a clear graphical representation of the positioning of the user's corpus data along these dimensions following the analysis, including comparison of the user's corpus position with those of Biber's (1989) text types.

MAT tokenises the data (i.e. it determines individual words and punctuation within a text), the results of which are then counted to determine the overall corpus size. This information is provided for both the dentistry and general medical corpora in Tables 2.1 and 2.2.

5. https://notepad-plus-plus.org/download/v7.5.9.html

6. https://sites.google.com/site/multidimensionaltagger/

Table 2.1 Dentistry research corpus – word tokens / type-token ratios

Journal title	Word tokens	TTR (per 400 tokens)
Acta Odontologica Scandinavica	29,605	211.40
British Dental Journal	32,749	201.60
Inter. Journal of Paediatric Dentistry	25,292	201.10
Journal of American Dental Assoc.	30,689	212.10
Journal of Canadian Dental Health Assoc.	21,088	217.40
Journal of Dental Biomechanics	30,104	202.40
Journal of Dental Research	25,767	206.10
Journal of Dentistry	38,149	207.10
Journal of Periodontology	34,009	190.40
Journal of Prosthetic Dentistry	29,751	200.40
Total	297,203	205.00

Table 2.2 General medical research corpus – word tokens / type-token ratios

Journal title	Word tokens	TTR (per 400 tokens)
Annals of Internal Medicine	41,035	208.30
British Medical Journal	28,514	204.10
Journal of American Medical Assoc.	42,388	201.20
Journal of Clinical Investigation	58,500	216.10
Journal of Bone and Joint Surgery	37,397	194.90
The Lancet	82,383	193.20
Medical Care	39,552	214.00
Nature	47,645	227.50
New England Journal of Medicine	36,598	201.90
PLOS Medicine	52,815	203.30
Total	466,827	206.45

It is apparent that articles produced for the dentistry discipline are much shorter, on the whole, than those written for general medical purposes. Based on the running text remaining following the cleaning procedure, the average article length within the dentistry corpus is 2,972 tokens, while the average article length in the general medical corpus is 4,669 tokens. Studies in *The Lancet*, *Journal of Clinical Investigation* and *PLOS Medicine* appear to be much longer than those in other journals. However, the statistics produced under MAT for the MDA analysis are normalised to n=100 tokens, and so the data across both dentistry and general medical corpora are still comparable despite their difference in size.

As another measure of comparability, MAT also calculates the type-token ratio (TTR) of individual texts by dividing the types (the total number of different words) occurring in a text by its tokens (the total number of words). A high TTR is indicative of a high degree of lexical variation while a low TTR indicates the opposite. If our two corpora held significantly different TTR values, this may indicate that the register or genres of the two corpora may be significantly different, and thus less comparable. Given our focus on experimental, AIMRD-type research articles in both corpora, the TTR should theoretically be largely similar across the two corpora. MAT utilises a default 400 tokens to calculate the type-token ratio, a benchmark figure as also used in Biber (1988) as "a compromise between accuracy and number of texts that could be measured" (Nini, 2015b: p. 29). This means the software counts the first 400 tokens of each text in the corpus, then outputs the number of unique types within those first 400 tokens as a rough measure of lexical variation for that corpus. We also used this benchmark to determine TTR between our two corpora, given the reported differences in corpus size above. The average TTR of the dentistry corpus was 205/400, while the average TTR of the general medical corpus was 206.50/400. This finding therefore suggests no significant difference between the two corpora in terms of this particular measure of lexical density, and is further evidence that the two corpora are suitable for comparison (at least, as far as the first 400 tokens of these articles are concerned).

2.4 MAT analyses across Biber's (1988) dimensions

Figure 2.1 describes the results of the MAT analysis of the linguistic features of both dentistry and general medical corpora as measured against Biber's (1988) dimensions and Biber's (1989) text types.[7] The five dimensions are shown on the x-axis (1 to 5), with the dimension scores (+/−) for our corpora and Biber's (1989) text types shown on the y-axis.

At first glance, the two corpora hold similar positions along the five dimensions represented in Figure 2.1, with text type scores along each dimension closest to those of 'scientific exposition' as one might expect from the genre in question (research articles in the sciences). The standardised z-scores for both corpora along Dimension 1 (involved vs. informational discourse) are slightly in the negative range, indicative of many nouns, long words and adjectives within the corpora. For Dimension 2 (narrative vs. non-narrative concerns), scores are again slightly in the negative, suggesting infrequent use of past tense and third person pronouns. For Dimension 3 (explicit vs. situation dependent reference) the scores for both our dentistry and general medical corpora are in fact higher than any other text

7. Nini's MAT tagger also outputs very useful figures with information for all of Biber's text types on them, but they are difficult to scale to the page – for this reason, we have produced our own figure with only 4 of Biber's text types shown in comparison to our two corpora.

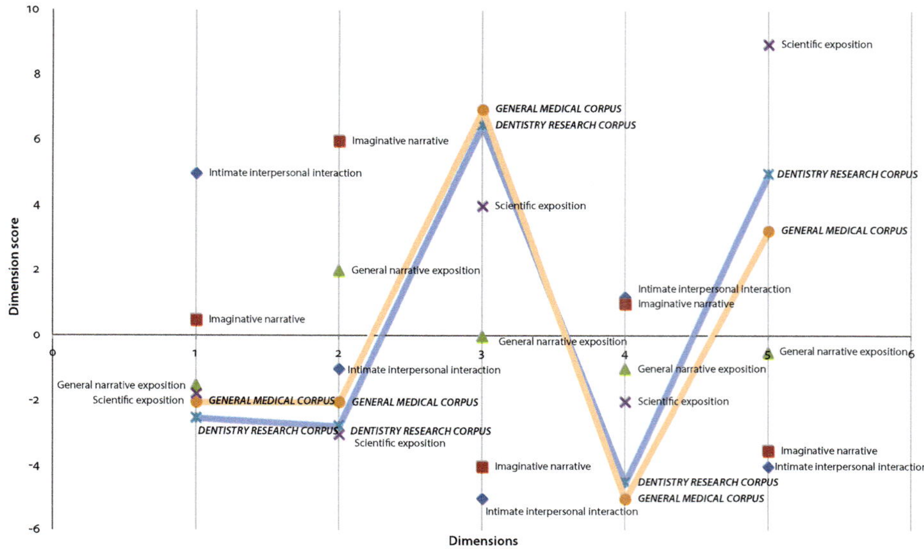

Figure 2.1 Dentistry and general medical corpus MDA results, shown against Biber's (1988) dimensions and (1989) text types

type – more so that 'scientific discourse' – which is indicative of a very high frequency of nominalisations. Both corpora have low scores along Dimension 4 (overt expression of persuasion). Text types with high scores on this dimension generally use linguistic features that explicitly mark the author's point of view and where the author frequently makes assessments of likelihood/certainty (e.g. strong presence of modal verbs and lexical 'hedges' or 'boosters', Hyland, 2005). Our corpora, therefore, are less likely to contain such features, suggesting the authors of these experimental research articles are presenting their statements and claims as facts. Finally, z-scores along Dimension 5 (abstract vs. non-abstract information) are in the slightly positive range for both corpora, suggestive of technical, formal writing containing frequent passive clauses and conjuncts.

There is, however, one significant source of variation between the dentistry and general medical corpora along Biber's (1988) dimensions, namely Dimension 5 (abstract vs non-abstract information). We conducted Mann-Whitney U analysis for each of the five dimensions (adjusted alpha = .01),[8] finding that the positioning of the dentistry corpus is significantly higher along Dimension 5 than that of the

8. When conducting multiple statistical tests on the same dataset, one must make corrections to avoid the possibility of 'data dredging/fishing' for statistical significance (e.g. Young & Karr, 2011).

general medical corpus ($U = 2{,}790$, $z = -5.399$, $p < .001$, $r = -.382$).[9] To investigate further, we then converted the normalised frequencies of all 81 linguistic features derived from the MAT analysis[10] to standardised z-scores in the *Statistical Package for the Social Sciences* (SPSS, version 20), then ran a multiple regression on these scores to determine which of these features were the most likely to be grouped along Dimension 5. The model used 7 iterations ($F [7, 192] = 4{,}316{,}157$, adjusted $r^2 = 1$) with the features isolated 100% predictive of this dimension. The features isolated were conjuncts (CONJ, $p < .001$), agentless passives (PASS, $p < .001$), adverbial subordinators (such as 'since', 'while', 'whereas', 'as soon as', and 'whereby', OSUB, $p < .001$) and past participle relatives with the wh-component deleted (e.g. 'the solution [which was] produced by this process', WZPAST, $p < .001$). Also in the model were wh-determiners (WDT, $p = .011$), emphatics (such as 'just', 'really', 'a lot', EMPH, $p = .039$) and place adverbials (such as 'above', 'alongside', 'below', 'beside', PLACE, $p = .043$). The normalised frequencies (per 100 tokens) are shown in Figure 2.2.

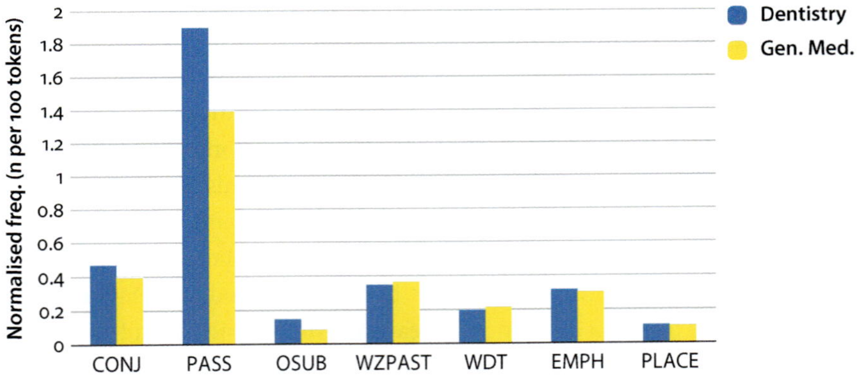

Figure 2.2 Normalised frequencies of linguistic features indicative of Dimension 5 across corpora

The dentistry corpus has a significantly higher frequency of passives (PASS, $U = 2{,}721$, $t = -5.569$, $p < .001$, $r = -.394$) and adverbial subordinators (OSUB, $U = 3{,}703$, $t = -3.171$, $p = .002$, $r = -.224$) than seen in the general medical corpus. Regarding the use of passives, dentistry research papers appear to contain very dense, detailed descriptions of procedures written entirely in the passive, often

9. Pearson R effect size interpretation, .10 = 'small', .30 = 'medium', .50 = 'large', .70 = 'very large', Cohen (1988).

10. A complete list of the features involved can be found in Nini's (2015b) manual for MAT.

with two or more passive constructions in the same sentence as exemplified in this passage from an article in *Acta Odontologica Scandinavica:*

> The method of specimen preparation and loading was adopted from Butz et al. (15). Forty caries-free, undamaged human maxillary central incisors were divided into 4 groups (group size of n/10) on the basis of cervical size. To ensure an even distribution of the size of teeth within the specimen groups, mesio-distal (MD) and facial-lingual (FL) dimensions were measured at the level of the cemento-enamel junction (CEJ). A size assessment value was calculated from the product of MD/FL. Teeth of extreme size were excluded and specimens were randomly distributed into test groups (Table I).

Papers in the general medical corpus, while still using passives frequently when compared to that of the other text types shown in Figure 2.2, tended to recount methodological procedures in active voice using past simple tense, as exemplified in this passage from a paper in *The Lancet* dealing with the creation of a statistical model:

> We modelled the prevalence of obesity as a fraction of the joint category of overweight and obesity. We used this method to ensure that the prevalence of obesity did not exceed the joint category of overweight and obesity, which is bound between 0 and 1. We explored the use of other covariates to predict prevalence, including average income per person and various measures of diet composition. Our results were not sensitive to the choice of these covariates and we present estimates based on the most parsimonious model. The appendix shows details on the various model specifications that we included.

For other adverbial subordinators, we used *AntConc* (Version 3.4.4, Anthony, 2014) to analyse the frequencies of the subordinators taken from a list in Nini's (2015b) MAT manual, then used Rayson's (2016) freely available *Log-likelihood Calculator*[11] to work out which, if any, of these subordinators were particularly associated with the dentistry corpus. In corpus linguistic terms, we are interested in whether any of these subordinators are *keywords* – that is, whether they are specifically associated with one corpus (here, our dentistry corpus) as compared with that of a reference corpus (here, the general medical corpus). This methodology requires the calculation of a statistical measure called log-likelihood (LL) which is used to determine the extent of the significance of that association -or *keyness* – of the phrase in question to the corpus in question. Log-likelihood (LL) is a contingency value representing potential significant differences between target wordings and non-target wordings across two or more corpora. This also provides a measure of effect size for the LL significance value in the form of the Bayes Information Criterion (BIC) measure (Wilson, 2013). This value is a measure of the strength of significant LL

11. http://ucrel.lancs.ac.uk/llwizard.html

p values in terms of degrees of evidence against the null hypothesis (i.e. the LL *p* value has no measurable effect), with scores varying between 0–2: low effect, 2–6: positive evidence against the null hypothesis (H0), 6–10: strong evidence against H0, > 10: very strong evidence against H0.

We found the dentistry papers made more frequent use of the adverbial subordinators 'while' (186 times in the dentistry corpus compared with 134 in the general medical corpus, LL = 48.14, $p < .0001$, BIC = 34.60) and 'whilst' (17 times in the dentistry corpus compared with zero hits in the general medical corpus, LL = 32.10, $p < .0001$, BIC = 18.56). We see that 'while' and 'whilst' are often used when elaborating on findings in the results sections of dentistry research articles, as with these examples from a paper in *Acta Odontologica Scandinavica*:

> All subjects but two had detectable levels of salivary mutans streptococci at baseline, while all exhibited growth of salivary lactobacilli.
>
> During the test periods with the probiotic test yogurt consumption, 8 subjects exhibited decreased scores (1–2 steps), 10 subjects had unchanged scores, while one displayed a 1-step increased score.
>
> After the test yogurt, decreased lactobacilli levels (1 score) were found in 7 subjects, while 2 subjects displayed increased scores.

In summary, our analysis in this section has revealed significant differences between the two corpora along the dimension of (non)abstract information. Specifically, dentistry research articles make much heavier use of the passive voice compared with research articles from the general medical field, while frequent use of the adverbial subordinators 'while' or 'whilst' when reporting experimental results is also a feature specific to dentistry research articles.

2.5 MDA Version 2: The functional dimensions of dentistry research articles

The previous MDA used pre-set linguistic dimensions sourced from Biber's (1988) work, which, as mentioned, are constitutive of a range of registers and text types. More specific analyses require the derivation and categorisation of the functional dimensions present within the target corpus itself, namely our corpus of dentistry research articles. To this end, we performed an exploratory factor analysis (EFA) on the 81 linguistic features isolated by the MAT tagger. An EFA is a statistical method used to describe variability among observed, correlated variables to derive a range of potentially unobserved variables called factors, which constitute the functional 'dimensions' that characterise that genre or register. The EFA in this chapter was conducted using the freely available JASP statistical program (Version 0.8.4).[12] The

12. https://jasp-stats.org/download/

software is constantly updated with new features and is compatible with a wide range of operating systems, and is generally more user friendly than SPSS and R when conducting EFA.

The form of EFA conducted was that of a direct oblimin rotation, which is classed as an oblique form of rotation. Rotation in EFA is the process involved in interpreting the factor matrices to arrive at a solution with the best simple structure. An oblique rotation allows for the possibility that the factors may be correlated, and this correlation can be ascertained statistically. We entered the original 81 linguistic features into the model, then began the process of eliminating individual features with low communality (i.e. variance in each item is explained by the extracted factors) and, in most cases, very low frequency in the corpus data as well. This process reduced the number of linguistic features present in the final model to 41 (see Appendix A for this list).

The final model resulted in a five-factor solution, based on the eigenvalues for these factors being greater than 1 (Kaiser, 1960) and analysis of the scree-plot (Cattell, 1966). Eigenvalues result from linear transformation that occurs during the EFA, and the larger the value, the stronger the derived factor in the model. The scree plot in Figure 2.3 displays the eigenvalues in graphical form, and the factors with highest eigenvalues are displayed on the left-hand side of the chart, dropping down the y-axis as the eigenvalues decrease for each factor. When analysing the scree plot, the researcher counts the number of factors on the chart that occur before the line drawn between them becomes near-horizontal, typically when the factor eigenvalues are equal to 1 (the rest of the factors on the line at this point are too weak to enter the model and are termed 'scree', hence the name 'scree plot').

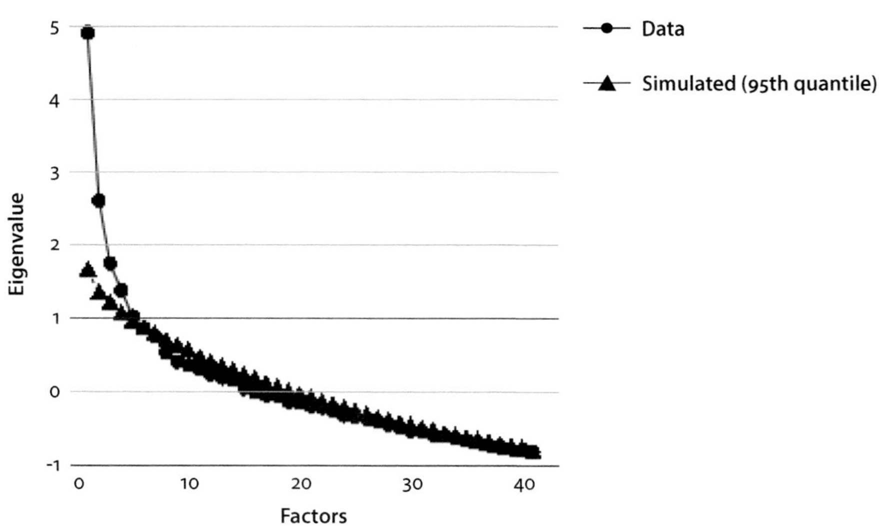

Figure 2.3 Scree plot for EFA

While both the eigenvalue > 1 and scree plot are useful for the researcher in working out how many factors should form the final model, they are both subjective measures of goodness-of-fit. To counter this, JASP reports three values generated from the model as additional statistical measures of goodness-of-fit. The first is that of the chi-squared value. For our model, the chi-squared value was $X^2 = 629.98$, d.f. = 625, p = .437. The non-significance of the chi-squared value is important because our null hypothesis is that there is no difference between the observed data and our hypothesized factor model, that is to say the factors explain the observed data, which is the case here. The second value generated by JASP is termed the *Root Mean Square Error of Approximation* (RMSEA), which is a goodness-of-fit index value that estimates the discrepancy between the model and the data per degree of freedom for the model. The RMSEA for our model was 0.048, where values less than .05 constitute a 'good' fit (Browne & Cudeck, 1992) and with values greater than .05 resulting in a weaker goodness-of-fit. The third value generated by JASP is that of the Tucker-Lewis Index (TLI), which is classed as a comparative fit index based on confirmatory factor analysis comparison of the chi-squared value of the implied matrix with that of a null model (the most typical being that all observed variables are uncorrelated), and with a value of 1 indicative of a 'perfect' fit. The TLI value from our model is .99, where values of > .95 are the cut-off for good fit (Hu & Bentler, 1998). Given that our five-factor model has surpassed the criteria for goodness-of-fit along these three measures, we are confident of the validity of the final model.

The final model is shown in Table 2.3, with the factor loading value displayed for each feature/factor. A factor loading cut-off value of >. 04 is commonly used for including a feature within a factor for both positive and negative factor loadings. Positive loadings denote a high frequency of a given feature within a given factor, while a negative loading denotes a low frequency of a feature within a factor.

We now attempt to define each factor by function. One issue is that the first two factors do not have significant negative loadings. These may be interpreted as 'functions' rather than 'dimensions'. For the purposes of interpretation, a 'dimension' implies a continuum of opposing features along which a given text will lie, while a 'function' implies a set of correlated features that may be present or absent in a given text without necessarily requiring an opposing set of features that have the inverse function. We have named the factors as either 'functions' or 'dimensions' accordingly.

Table 2.3 Final EFA model of the dentistry corpus

Feature	Factor 1	Factor 2	Factor 3	Factor 4	Factor 5
Predictive modals (PRMD)	0.751				
Verbs-Base form (VB)	0.686				
Demonstrative pronouns (DEMP)	0.644				
Conditional adverbial subordinators (COND)	0.475				
WH-clauses (WHCL)	0.423				
WH-Pronoun (WP)		0.924			
WH relative clauses on subject position (WHSUB)		0.89			
Second person pronouns (SPP2)		0.419			
Verbs-past tense (VBD)			0.815		
Pro Verb DO (PROD)			0.408		
WH-determiner (WDT)			−0.477		
Verb-present tense (VPRT)			−0.815		
Passives (PASS)				0.94	
Verb-past participle (VBN)				0.85	
Third person pronoun (TPP3)				−0.46	
Perfect aspect (PEAS) (e.g. HAVE + VBD, VBN)					0.593
Coordinating Conjunction (CC)					0.449
Nouns (not nominalisation or gerund) (NN)					−0.466
Adjectives (JJ)					−0.566

2.5.1 Function 1 – Confirming findings as facts

The first factor primarily involves the use of predictive modals (*will, would, shall*) in combination with verbs in their base form. In the introduction or literature review sections of many of the articles in the dentistry corpus, these two features are used to add legitimacy and certainty to claims made about previous findings in the literature. This works as a booster (Hyland, 2005) that strengthens the proposition as a whole, rather than the kind of tentative, hedged claims that would be made through possibility modals such as *may, might,* and *could.* This is shown in the following example from the *Journal of Dental Biomechanics*:

> Studies have been done to address the mechanical deficiencies by adding reinforcing agents to the materials. However, reinforcing agents or fillers will increase the rigidity or Young's modulus of a maxillofacial material. Young's Modulus is the slope of the elastic region in a stress-strain curve and is conventional referred to as the stiffness of a material. Increasing the modulus will decrease the flexibility of the prosthesis and processability of the uncured resin. One such example is the addition of nylon material to the silicone material to make the prostheses more durable [2].

The use of the conditional adverbial subordinators *if* and *unless* also accompany the use of predictive modals to provide elaboration on possible circumstances involved in claims about previous findings, as with this example from the *Journal of Periodontology*:

> For 1-piece non-submerged implants [4, 7, 8] or 2-stage implants used with a single-stage non-submerged protocol, the biologic width will form at the time of implant placement. This phenomenon is not related to loading and it will occur whether the implant is unloaded or loaded [7]. The biologic rationale is that the bone exposed to the oral cavity will always cover itself with periosteum and connective tissue. Additionally, connective tissue will always cover itself with epithelium. If a chronic irritant, such as bacteria, reaches the implant abutment interface through screw-access channels [9-12], or if the abutment is removed after initial healing [6], the bone will resorb to create a distance from this chronically exposed or irritated area.

Demonstrative pronouns are also commonly used while discussing claims made in previous studies, referring directly to findings summarised in previous clauses before the author makes their claim about those findings. This is shown in the following example from the *Journal of Dentistry*:

> Whilst rates of edentulism are falling in most Western countries population demographics are changing; as people live longer there will be an increasing proportion of people in the older age group, the group most likely to need dentures [10–12]. Despite this, it does seem likely that the absolute number of people who need complete dentures in the developed world will decrease over the next few decades but this will still leave a substantial number of edentulous patients requiring treatment In the UK this is likely to be half the number required at the end of 1999.

As previously mentioned, we do not have negative loadings of any features on this factor and so can only assume that papers/journals that lack this confirming/boosting function will have negative standardized z-scores for this factor. The *Journal of the American Dental Association* has quite a high positive score for this factor (z = 3.20) suggesting that articles within this journal frequently employ this function, while only the *Journal of Dentistry* has a low (although not significantly so) negative score (z = – 1.04).

2.5.2 Function 2 – Categorising patient types

For the second factor, WH-pronouns ('what', 'who' and 'whom') and WH-relative clauses on subject position (e.g. 'the man who likes popcorn') are frequently used in a number of texts in the dentistry corpus to categorise and elaborate on the conditions of patients as described in the research. This function is most commonly found in the methodology section, as with this example from the *Journal of the American Dental Association*:

> We queried the electronic medical record system used by the USC School of Dentistry (Axium, Exan Academic, Port Coquitlam, British Columbia, Canada) to determine the number of active patients who had a history of alendronate use. We then identified all patients receiving alendronate at the time of the study or in the past who also were being treated for active ONJ in the Oral Surgery clinic [...]. All patients with ONJ who we included in the study had radiographic evidence of an ill-defined lytic lesion of the jawbone in addition to clinical evidence of exposed necrotic bone (sequestra) with mucosal ulceration (Figure). [...] We also queried the electronic medical record system to identify all patients (those who received and did not receive alendronate) who had undergone tooth extraction – the most common dental procedure associated with ONJ development postoperatively – or had planned to do so.

The *British Dental Journal* is most closely associated with this function (z = 3.80), while journals with relatively low or negative scores are *Acta Odontologica Scandinavica* (z = – 1.70) and *International Journal of Paediatric Dentistry* (z = – 1.40).

2.5.3 Dimension 1 – Narrative vs. non-narrative concerns

The third factor is largely similar to that of Biber's (1988) Dimension 2, and we have kept Biber's label for that dimension here. Texts with high z-scores along this dimension are rich in past tense verbs as opposed to frequent use of present tense verbs in texts with low z-scores. Past tense verbs feature heavily in the literature review, methodology (as passives), results, and discussion (as passives) sections, as with these examples all taken from the same paper published in *Acta Odontologica Scandinavica*:

> [Literature review] Three previous studies reported In-Ceram crown survival rates of 98.4% to 100%, with maximum follow-up periods of 24 to 56 months. [25,27,29] However, those studies had small sample sizes (n = 61 to 63) [...]. Another anecdotal study reported only 2 losses among 352 In-Ceram crowns placed over a 5-year period, but the methods and follow-up rate were not reported [28]. In contrast, a study of 35 In-Ceram crowns studied for 2.5 to 21 months reported that 3 crowns fractured after 4, 8, and 12 months [26]. Survival rates at fixed intervals were not reported, but the failure rate was probably an order of magnitude greater than found in the other reports.
>
> [Methodology] For the first 3 years, all the laboratory procedures were performed by the treating dentist according to manufacturer guidelines. [32–34] For the later years, most of the copings were fabricated by a single certified dental technician. Core thicknesses of at least 0.5 mm were used. Where interocclusal space allowed,

> 0.7-mm core thicknesses were used for molar teeth. Core thickness was checked with spring calipers before veneering with porcelain.
>
> [Results] Two patients died and 9 patients were lost to follow-up before termination of the study. [...] . Of the patients successfully followed to the termination of the study, approximately 73% were examined in the office and the other 27% who had not attended the office in the 6 months before study termination completed the telephone survey. The general dentists currently caring for the telephone-surveyed patients reported no previously undocumented In-Ceram failures, and verified **the** data provided by the patients' telephone surveys
>
> [Discussion] This study had many limitations. Only complete crowns were included and success rates of other types of crowns were not reported. All clinical procedures were performed by a single clinician, so selection biases may have been introduced.

The use of 'did' as a main verb also contributes towards the narrative reporting of events as they unfolded, as with these examples from a paper in the *Journal of Dental Biomechanics*:

> In the 1.5-mm mucosal model, the magnetic attachments showed significantly lower bending moments than did the ball attachment
> On the other hand, the cushion type reportedly had little effect on the denture displacement and exhibited lower lateral stresses than did the flat type [14]

However, certain papers use present tense verbs to describe methodological procedures that actually took place in the past, eschewing a narrative retelling of events for a more instructional approach. This example, also from *Journal of Dental Biomechanics*, highlights the use of present tense verbs for this purpose:

> In each photo 15 points are selected, as seen in Figure 1(a). Five points are along the wall on the right-hand side wall, 5 points along the left-hand side (gingival) wall, and 5 points along the bottom. The points are all plotted on a 2-dimensional Cartesian (x,y) coordinate system as shown in Figure 1(b). Each corner has a radius, and the points are selected just outside the radius. Along each wall the two endpoints are selected first. The spreadsheet suggests approximately where the middle three points should be. For example, the right wall **is** mostly vertical. Therefore, using the y-coordinates from the two endpoints, the spreadsheet will give three more y-coordinates equally spaced between the endpoints. The user attempts to find the three middle points along the wall with y-coordinates that are within 0.01 mm of the suggested y-coordinate. This process ensures that all five points along a given wall are nearly equally distanced.

Present tense verbs are also frequently used in some papers to describe the clinical features of dental problems in patients, as with this example from the *Journal of the Canadian Dental Health Association* about cherubism, a form of bone lesion in children:

> Affected children are normal at birth and are without clinically or radiographically evident disease until 14 months to 3 years of age. At that time, symmetric enlargement of the jaws begins. Typically, the earlier the lesion appears, the more rapidly it progresses. The self-limited bone growth usually begins to slow down when the patient reaches 5 years of age, and stops by the age of 12 to 15 years [10,11].

WH-determiners such as 'which' are used to describe the clinical features of dental problems, as with this example also from the *Journal of the Canadian Dental Health Association* about bipolar disorder, in a paper about how dentists can provide therapy for this condition:

> Manic episodes are characterized by hyperactivity, which may involve excessive participation in multiple activities (e.g., sexual, occupational, religious or political). There is often a demanding and increasing nature to these activities of which the individual is unaware. [...] Both manic and depressive episodes result in significant impairment in social and occupational functioning, which can lead to marital instability, alienation from family and loss of employment [3].

Despite the TTR ratio of the journals within the corpus being largely similar, it is important to consider individual variation in terms of the relative positioning of each journal along a given linguistic dimension. Figure 2.4 describes the z-score position for each journal in the dentistry corpus along our Dimension 1.

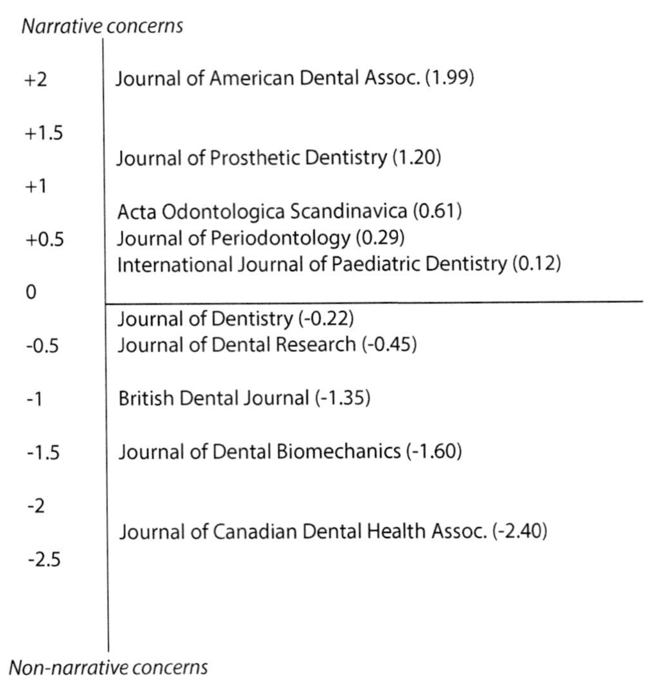

Figure 2.4 Narrative vs. non-narrative concerns among RAs in top dentistry journals

There is clearly significant variation along this dimension among the different dental journals, with the *Journal of the American Dental Association* more narrative in style than most other journals in this field (+ 1.99). The *Journal of Canadian Dental Health Association* is less likely to use a narrative, past tense-filled reportage (– 2.40), as already seen in the previously quoted examples.

2.5.4 Dimension 2 – Active vs. passive

Factor 4 involves the use of passive constructions (PASS, VBN) at the positive end of this dimension, with third person pronouns (TPP3) involved in active voice constructions featuring at the negative end. As mentioned already, the passive is a very frequently used construction in dentistry research articles, and is used across a number of sections within the paper including the methodology, results and discussion sections, as shown here from a paper in *Journal of Prosthetic Dentistry*:

> [Methodology] For the first 3 years, all the laboratory procedures were performed by the treating dentist according to manufacturer guidelines. [32–34] For the later years, most of the copings were fabricated by a single certified dental technician. Core thicknesses of at least 0.5 mm were used. Where interocclusal space allowed, 0.7-mm core thicknesses were used for molar teeth. Core thickness was checked with spring calipers before veneering with porcelain.
>
> [Results] For the 223 crowns in 53 patients with at least 36 months of follow-up, survival curves were compared with respect to crown placement on anterior, premolar, or molar teeth (Fig. 4). Although no statistical difference was discerned (P > .05), anterior crowns (n = 97) tended to have a slightly higher 3-year survival rate (97.9%) than for premolars (n = 36, survival rate = 93.5%) or for molars (n = 64, survival = 93.8%) (Fig. 4). Survival curves were compared for crowns in male patients (n = 53) versus crowns in female patients (n = 170), but no difference was found (both had 3-year survival rates of approximately 96%) (P > .05). Survival curves were also compared for crowns in patients showing signs of excessive wear or bruxing (n = 53) versus without such signs (n = 170), but no difference was found.

However, there are numerous occasions when active voice constructions with third-person pronouns are used to describe methodological procedures involving the actions of the authors as active participants in the unfolding events, as well as to refer to the dentists themselves. This is exemplified in a passage from the *Journal of American Dental Association*:

> The authors requested a list of 4,970 randomly chosen general practitioners from the American Dental Association Survey Center. They then sent those dentists a written survey asking whether and in what numbers they treat children; the ages and caries levels of any children they do treat; their perceptions of their educational experiences in paediatric dentistry, and their perceived needs for continuing education in paediatric dentistry. They analyzed data using $X^{2.}$

The use of these third-person pronouns also appears to feature in studies where questionnaires were administered, as with this example from the *British Dental Journal*:

> Interestingly, the majority of parents (78%) reported that they would like to have access to more tooth brushing programmes in schools and nurseries in their area. Also, 68% percent of them thought that an oral health programme in the hospital would be helpful. Half of the parents thought training one of their peers from their local community to give oral health advice would be helpful, and 30% thought home visits from dental professionals would be helpful. Only 11% said they would like help finding another dentist. Only one parent said we should do nothing (Fig.3).

Figure 2.5 describes the relative position of each journal along the continuum of passive to active. Again, the *Journal of the American Dental Assoc.* stands in contrast to most other journals in the corpus, scoring very low along this dimension, with

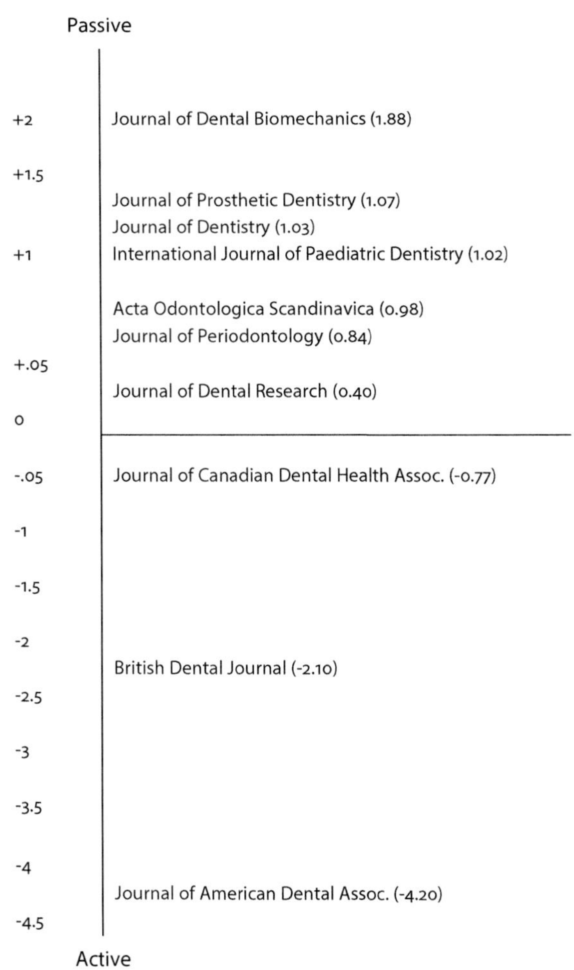

Figure 2.5 Active vs. passive features among research articles in top dentistry journals

the *British Dental Journal* also scoring low. Journals more focused on specific procedures such as *Journal of Dental Biomechanics* and *Journal of Prosthetic Dentistry* tended to score higher on this dimension than other journals, utilising a high frequency of passives for detailed descriptions of said procedures.

2.5.5 Dimension 3 – Involved vs. informational discourse

The fifth factor identified in the EFA involves the use of the perfect (HAVE + VBN, VBD) at the positive end of the continuum for this dimension, with nouns at the negative end. This is similar to Biber's (1988) Dimension 1 'involved vs. informational discourse', with 'involved discourse' being more affective and interactional (containing more verbs and pronouns) than 'informational discourse', which is closer to that of academic prose (containing more nouns and adjectives). We have decided to keep Biber's label for our Dimension 3. In our corpus, the use of the perfect is common when describing previous findings in literature review sections, as with these examples all taken from a single paper in *Journal of Canadian Dental Assoc.:*

> Studies have found a correlation between low vitamin C intake and the presence of an oral lesion [13].
>
> Numerous studies have examined the transformation rates of oral leukoplakias – that is, the time that elapses before a leukoplakic lesion shows malignant change.
>
> It has been observed that the oral cancers due to smokeless tobacco use may occur in sites that are different from the cancers caused by other factors.
>
> Studies have shown that the presence of dysplastic changes cannot be predicted by the habit or by the clinical grading of the lesion. [28,29]
>
> Individual cases of ANUG, gingivitis and periodontitis have been reported [30], but a clear relationship does not exist between a generalized periodontal condition and smokeless tobacco use. [8,31]
>
> Gingival recession and attachment loss have been shown to occur in the area adjacent to where the smokeless tobacco is held [31–34]

The main reporting verbs (find, examine, observe, report, etc.) represent an active, involved situation for the inanimate subjects that precede them, indicative of a more dynamic, ongoing narration style. Another common use of the perfect in the dentistry corpus is that of hedging predictions about events that the authors do not yet have firm answers for, such as with these examples from *Journal of American Dental Assoc:*

> The necrotic tooth no. 27, which was treated subsequently with endodontic therapy, also may have been a risk factor for osteonecrosis of the jaw in this case
>
> Although the dentist did not remove bone and used a low resistance setting, the interproximal bone may have been affected thermally by its close proximity to the operating current.

At the other end of the dimension – that of informational discourse – a dense combination of nouns and adjectives are used to clearly denote specific factors and symptoms involved in dental problems, as with this abstract taken from the *Journal of Dental Research:*

> The eventual outcome of dental caries is determined by the dynamic balance between pathological factors that lead to demineralization and protective factors that lead to remineralization. Pathological factors include acidogenic bacteria, inhibition of salivary function, and frequency of ingestion of fermentable carbohydrates. Protective factors include salivary flow, numerous salivary components, antibacterials (both natural and applied), fluoride from extrinsic sources, and selected dietary components.

Figure 2.6 describes where each journal in the dentistry corpus falls along this dimension. Overall, the level of variation shown along this dimension is less than that of the other two dimensions, although the more general *British Dental Journal* has the highest positive score along the involved pole, while the research focused *Journal of Dental Research* has the highest negative score along the informational pole.

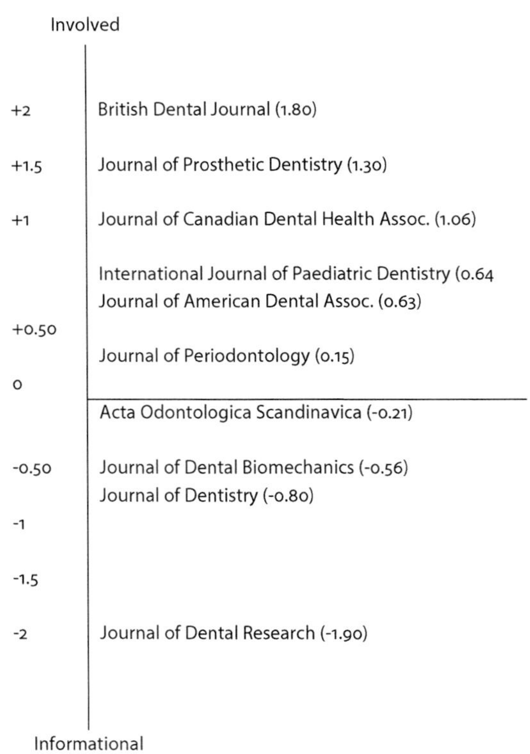

Figure 2.6 Involved vs. informational discourse within RAs from top dentistry journals

2.5.6 Dentistry vs. General medical research reports

The final part of the analysis involved the comparison of the z-scores for each function / dimension across each text in the dentistry and general medical corpora, so as to ascertain inter-corpus variation along the five factors identified. Five Mann-Whitney U tests were performed on the data (alpha = 0.01), one for each factor.

No significant differences were found across the two corpora for Function 1 (confirming findings as facts), with papers in both corpora just as likely to have this function ($U = 5{,}104$, $z = -.254$, $p = .799$). There were also no significant differences found across the two corpora for Dimension 1 (narrative vs. non-narrative concerns, $U = 5{,}881$, $z = 2.15$, $p = .031$ – insignificant after alpha correction) nor Dimension 3 (involved vs. informational discourse, $U = 4{,}767$, $z = -.569$, $p = .569$). Research articles in both dentistry and general medical fields utilise both narrative and non-narrative elements for different functions, with dentistry articles slightly more narrative in style overall and with general medical research reports slightly less so. The dentistry research articles were also slightly more 'involved' in the way that discourse is presented than the style seen in articles in the general medical corpus.

However, significant differences were found across corpora for Function 2 (categorising patient types), with test statistics of $U = 6{,}882$, $z = 4.60$, $p < .001$, $r = -.326$). The dentistry research articles had significantly lower median z-scores for this function that found in the general medical corpus. Here, we attribute this finding to an increased focus on patients in the general medical journals, rather than a focus on procedures as seen in the dentistry research articles. While all of the papers in the general medical corpus were research reports in the AIMRD format, the highly specialised, technical nature of experimental dental research has a much stronger focus on what was done rather than who it was done to, as evidenced by the lack of WH-pronouns and WH-relatives.

This non-personal characteristic of dentistry research writing is also confirmed by significant cross-corpus differences for Dimension 2 (active vs. passive), with the dentistry corpus found to have significantly higher z-scores along this dimension than the general medical corpus ($U = 3{,}285$, $z = -4.19$, $p < .001$, $r = -.303$). This can again be attributed to the very detailed procedural descriptions present in the methodology sections of dentistry reports as compared with those in the general medical field. Dentistry writers condense very complicated procedures into very tight sections of text, necessitating very frequent use of the passive construction with as many as two or three instances of this construction per sentence.

2.6 Discipline-specific lexis and phraseology

Following the MDA, we opted to determine the lexical choices specific to the dentistry corpus for the purposes of generating a teachable list of key vocabulary that could be used to generate future ESAP activities. Here, we again used *AntConc* to determine the keywords and their LL values from the dentistry corpus using the general medical corpus as the reference corpus for comparison, and using Rayson's *Log-Likelihood Calculator* to determine the Log-likelihood and BIC effect sizes of the keyness statistics. For negative scores, the BIC is read as 'in favour of' instead of 'against' the H0, and so wordings with significant LL values but negative BIC effect sizes are not included in the results.

In total, 912 keywords with an LL of over 15.13 (p < .0001) were specifically associated with the dentistry corpus, after the removal of all abbreviations, acronyms, proper names, mis-parsed words, symbols, certain common nouns that were considered as very likely to be non-discipline-specific (e.g. 'students', 'boy', 'girl', etc.), and function words (e.g. 'the', 'a', 'when', etc.) from the collated list. Table 2.4 represents only the top 50 keywords specific to the dentistry corpus; the full list of 912 keywords is included in Appendix B.

Table 2.4 Top 50 keywords in the dentistry corpus

Keyword	Freq. Dent.	Freq. Gen. Med.	LL	BIC	Keyword	Freq. Dent.	Freq. Gen. Med.	LL	BIC
dental	1,165	9	2089.46	2089.68	*molars*	146	0	273.97	262.16
teeth	721	5	1298.18	1293.16	*bonding*	146	1	262.99	251.17
tooth	699	7	1240.11	1234.81	*surfaces*	161	6	256.38	244.7
caries	586	3	1064.95	1058.34	*wear*	148	3	251.25	239.44
periodontal	386	1	711.41	702.44	*maxillary*	143	3	242.07	230.2
dentin	373	0	699.94	690.82	*occlusal*	129	0	242.07	230.06
enamel	336	2	607.98	602.13	*mandibular*	131	1	235.05	223.06
oral	541	93	578.87	571.05	*zirconia*	131	1	235.05	223.06
resin	324	6	553.97	544.22	*restoration*	156	10	227.09	215.32
restorations	261	0	489.77	479.32	*composite*	205	33	225.85	214.49
implant	305	11	487.77	477.76	*strength*	203	32	225.66	214.29
materials	305	14	471.32	461.3	*orthodontic*	116	0	217.67	205.51
etch	253	1	462.68	452.13	*fracture*	230	51	216.04	204.84
surface	379	51	448.68	439.24	*bracket*	115	0	215.79	203.62
dentine	223	0	418.46	407.56	*crown*	114	0	213.92	201.73
ceramic	246	7	404.54	393.86	*adhesives*	112	0	210.17	197.95
crowns	214	0	401.57	390.57	*wire*	117	1	209.01	196.85
adhesive	209	2	371.56	360.48	*incisal*	110	0	206.41	194.18

(continued)

Table 2.4 (*continued*)

Keyword	Freq. Dent.	Freq. Gen. Med.	LL	BIC	Keyword	Freq. Dent.	Freq. Gen. Med.	LL	BIC
bone	428	110	367.34	358.04	*width*	129	5	204.34	192.29
material	273	25	365.35	354.86	*rinse*	106	0	198.91	186.62
periodontitis	194	0	364.04	352.8	*shade*	106	0	198.91	186.62
bond	212	8	337.03	325.94	*force*	176	27	197.89	186.24
implants	211	8	335.23	324.13	*denture*	103	0	193.28	180.96
specimens	263	45	282.01	271.25	*dentition*	102	0	191.4	179.07
restorative	154	1	277.89	266.17	*hypodontia*	102	0	191.4	179.07

These keywords can be categorised as: *diseases and conditions*, including 'caries', 'wear', 'periodontitis', and 'hypodontia'; *substances and materials* including 'dentin', 'enamel', 'resin', 'dentine', 'ceramic', 'adhesive', 'bone', 'zirconia', and 'composite'; *locations and positions* including 'width', 'periodontal', 'surface', 'occlusal', 'mandibular', 'incisal' and 'dentition'; and *procedures*, including 'restoration', 'implant', 'etch', and 'bonding'.

Following this analysis, we then used an alternative keyword generator (*Scattertext*, Kessler, 2017)[13] that provides a visual representation of the keywords in both target and reference corpora at the same time (Figure 2.7). *Scattertext* uses a 'dense rank difference' method of determining corpus keyness in a visual output, with the x-axis indicating the rank of a word or bigram along this axis in the reference corpus, with the same for the target corpus along the y-axis. The most frequent terms, regardless of ties, are ranked first on each axis, the next most frequent terms, regardless of ties, are ranked second, etc. Terms more associated with a particular corpus are a further distance from the diagonal line between the lower-left and upper-right corners, while terms are also coloured according to this distance. Once the chart is generated, the visualisation is displayed in a HTML document, and users can actually click the 'dots' visible on the chart to display the corresponding word or phrase,[14] with some examples of that word or phrase shown in concordances from the corpus.

13. https://github.com/JasonKessler/scattertext

14. due to the large number of keywords generated, not all keywords are visible as text, but are displayed as dots instead which can then be clicked by the user to display them.

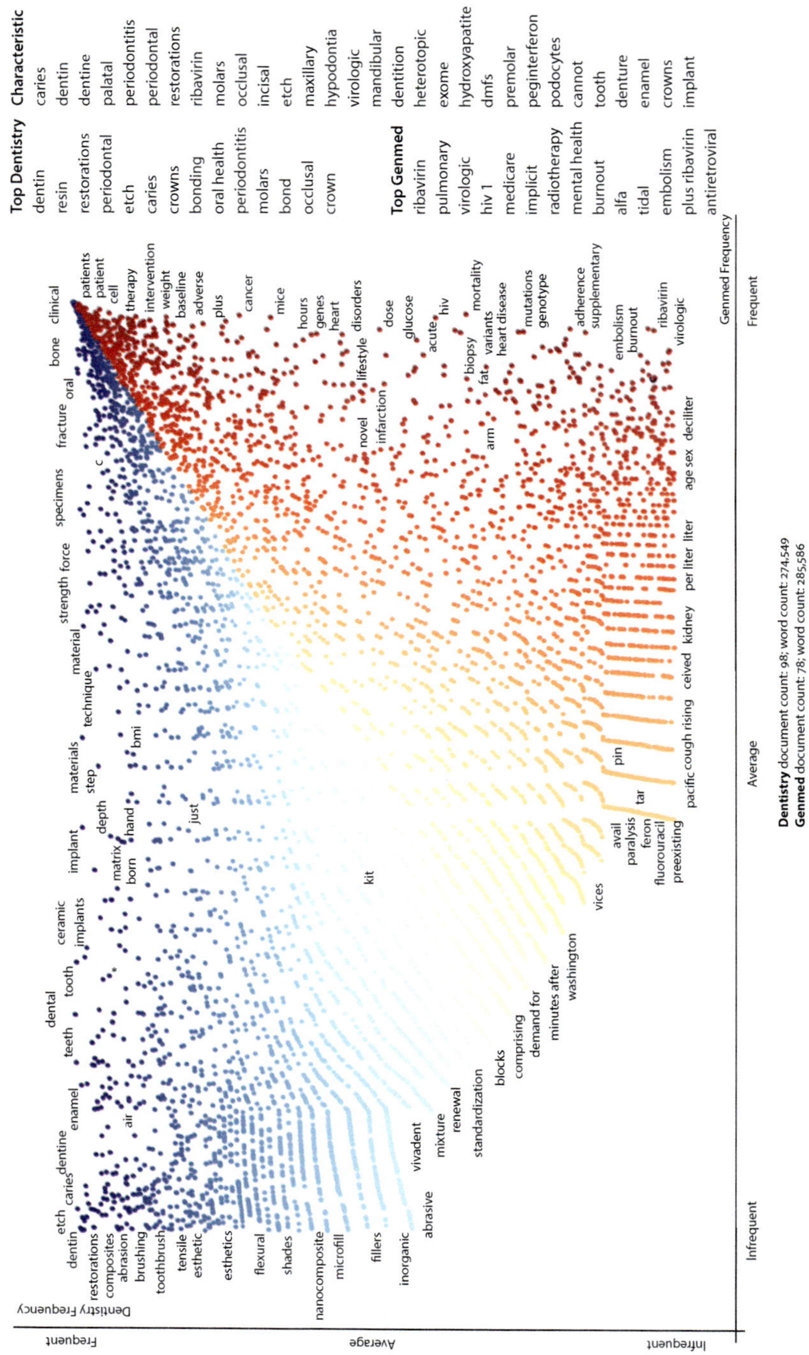

Figure 2.7 Keywords from the dentistry and general medical corpora using Scattertext (Kessler, 2017)

On the right-hand side of Figure 2.7, one can see the top keywords for the dentistry corpus, including 'dentin', 'resin', 'restorations', etc. as also seen in Table 4 above, as well as the top keywords from the general medical corpus, and a longer list of words generally representative of the dentistry corpus.

An additional analysis was then conducted to determine possible 2- and 3-word combinations (or *n-grams*) in our corpus, again using *AntConc*. Looking at 2-word compound nouns or nouns with adjectival modifiers, the list shown in Table 2.5 was derived, using a frequency cut-off of n = > 30 in the corpus as a whole. With only a few exceptions, these were all unique to the dentistry corpus and not also found in the general medical corpus[15].

Table 2.5 Top 2-gram noun compounds in the dentistry corpus

Expression	Frequency	Expression	Frequency
oral health	169	*third molars*	39
periodontal disease	159	*oral surgery*	38
self-etch	139	*smokeless tobacco*	38
bond strength	91	*fracture resistance*	37
dental caries	91	*hybrid layer*	37
mechanical properties	79	*etch adhesives*	36
in vitro	74	*implant placement*	36
risk factors	73	*dental arch*	35
long term	72	*primary care*	35
ceramic veneers	70	*tooth preparation*	34
dental school	63	*gap widths*	33
stem cells	63	*tobacco use*	33
bulk fill	61	*tooth brushing*	33
phosphoric acid	60	*anterior teeth*	32
dental treatment	57	*attachment loss*	30
tooth wear	48	*incisal edge*	30
sucking habits	47	*soft tissue*	30
control group	45		
elastic modulus	44		
dental health	43		
oral hygiene	42		
natural tooth	41		
shade guide	40		
smear layer	40		
cross sectional	39		

15. AntConc does not generate keyness statistics when using its n-gram function, so the frequency of these expressions and those in Table 6 were manually checked in the general medical corpus using AntConc.

Looking next at 3-word combinations in the dentistry corpus (Table 2.6), the data yielded a number of noun phrase stems of the form 'the [noun] of' along with other structural, interactive metadiscourse markers, for example 'with respect to'. These do not appear to be specific to dentistry (a similar list was also seen in the general medical corpus data) and so can be taken as typical of research papers generally. However, the list still represents a useful, teachable resource highly suitable for ESAP activities.

Table 2.6 Top 3-grams in the dentistry corpus

Expression	Frequency	Range	Expression	Frequency	Range
the presence of	85	44	*in relation to*	30	14
the results of	69	40	*the association between*	27	14
the prevalence of	63	21	*the development of*	26	23
the purpose of	40	33	*the importance of*	26	16
with respect to	40	20	*the absence of*	25	14
the fact that	39	24	*the need for*	25	16
the majority of	37	18	*the proportion of*	23	11
in accordance with	36	18	*the application of*	20	14
in order to	36	22	*the basis of*	20	16
the aim of	34	27	*the degree of*	20	14
the effects of	34	18	*the lack of*	20	15
the relationship between	33	17	*the management of*	20	8
by means of	32	18	*the percentage of*	20	12
when compared to	31	12			

2.7 Chapter summary

The findings in this chapter represent a teachable set of functional lexico-grammatical dimensions of experimental dentistry research papers, and lists of disciplinary lexis and phrases that frequently occur within the experimental research article genre generally and those that are specific to the dentistry discipline.

Both MDA analyses conducted in this chapter confirm the central role of the passive construction in dentistry research writing, and its use is not confined solely to the methodology section, but is also found in other sections of the article including the results and discussion. This has a major knock-on effect on the selection of verbs and their tense, pronominal forms, participles and a range other associated forms, and appears to be the main defining characteristic of dentistry research writing as compared with that of Biber's (1989) text types and of general medical research writing. Our data confirms a number of other studies investigating the role of the passive in science writing. Riley (1991) describes an expository function of the passive for recounting procedures and describing data, with active structures used for argumentative purposes such as critique of previous research or attempts to present new theories. Leong (2014) in his corpus study of passives in science writing found that passive constructions accounted for as much as 30% of all constructions, while Amdur, Kurwan and Morris (2010), in a similar corpus study on medical research articles, found the ratio of passive to active constructions as high as 50% in some papers. Leong explains the function of the passive in terms of the general goal of science to represent the world "in terms of objects, things, and materials" (c.f. Ding, 1998: p. 117) rather than humans, with Amdur et al. (2010: p. 109) suggesting that journal editors are the reason for its prevalence, suggesting "many medical articles are written to be published and cited, but not to be read". This is despite specialists on medical writing lamenting the passive as a construction that "reduces energy" or produces "sluggish academic prose" (Lingard, 2015: p. 53–54). It is apparent from our analysis, however, that despite a degree of variation among top journals in dentistry in the use of passive, the passive's pervasiveness in dentistry writing is not going away any time soon.

Arguments as to the source, history or future of the passive in dentistry writing aside, our findings have reconfirmed the importance of raising awareness of the passive and other constructions including past tense and the perfect to the novice writers on our ESAP course. This is not an easy task, with even those with a high proficiency of L2 English as well as novice L1 writers struggling to reproduce these conventionalised forms in their own writing (Holtzman, Elliot, Biber, & Sanders, 2005; Hinkel, 2004). Holtzman et al.'s (2005) study of L1 novice medical writers' articles found the percentage of sentences written in passive voice ranged from zero to 73 percent, and that overall the quality of writing was assessed at below the eleventh grade for comprehension, with some students at the level of middle school children. Swales and Feak (2000) suggest the way to overcome the issue for the passive voice is to direct students to learn by chunking certain verbs frequently associated with the passive voice (e.g. 'considered', 'found', 'used') as fixed, idiomatic expressions (e.g. 'it was considered that …'), which can be presented in the form of lists or built into grammar tasks. Likewise, our keyword and 2-, 3-gram lists derived from the analyses in this chapter lend themselves quite easily to "relatively simple" (Hinkel, 2004: p. 24) pedagogical treatment. We return to the pedagogical affordances generated from our analysis in Chapter 5, and evaluate the contribution of the findings of this chapter to our overall goals and those of the field in Chapter 7.

CHAPTER 3

Persuasive stories?

Professional and novice research reports for Dental Public Health

3.1 Introduction

As mentioned in Chapter 1, the dentistry discipline plays a highly visible role in the maintenance of public health within the local community where dentists practice. However, there is little literature discussing how professional dentistry writers report on Dental Public Health related research, with even less known about how novice disciplinary writers are able to report on their engagement with the public they eventually serve (Crawford, Adami, Johnson, Knight, Knoernschild, Obrez, Patson, Punwani, Zaki, & Licari, 2007). The goal of the writer in conveying research findings on Dental Public Health is less clinical and more persuasive in nature, as authors disseminating their research "*advocate* for public health policy, legislation, and regulations to protect and promote the public's oral health, and overall health" (Altman & Mascarenhas, 2016: p. s18, emphasis ours). Writers of Dental Public Health-related research need to appropriately balance the voices of 'practitioner' and 'researcher' with those of the 'reporter' and 'advocate', requiring those trained in Dental Public Health writing to "be proficient in communication [so] to interact effectively with multiple audiences" (Hernandez, Rosenstock & Gebbie, 2003: p. 8).

This requirement is currently met via discipline-specific English language support to the yearly cohort of approximately 70 students in year five of the degree. The new English-in-the-Discipline (ED) course was developed to enhance students' understanding of disciplinary research and allow them to acquire effective writing strategies for scientific report writing in the context of public health research, running parallel to the Faculty's compulsory module in that year, the Community Health Project (CHP), rather than in the freshman year, as it was pre-ED (see Chapter 5 for an overview as to this provision). Since 1984, dentistry students from different cohorts have conducted CHP projects on a wide selection of Dental Public Health issues to advance current knowledge of Hong Kong's specific oral health conditions and care provision. The CHP thus provides dentistry students a new learning opportunity to participate in project-based research activities, where 'knowledge is synthesized and transferred through the training process of planning, organizing, conducting, and presenting a community health project' (Faculty of Dentistry, 2015). The language features involved in the inextricable connection between language and content in presenting research findings are one of the key aspects of the ED course materials. In order to convince students of the value of taking on additional ESAP provision at such a late stage of their studies, there is a need for objective linguistic evidence that can reveal how soon-to-be graduates' academic writing differs from that of published disciplinary writing, that is, evidence outside of teachers' feedback and the grades on the CHP submissions. Such evidence could be used to provide future graduates the chance to critically reflect on the style and register used within their writing as compared with that used within the profession they hope to enter, while acknowledging that such writing is the main way of communicating with both their profession and the community they aim to serve.

We aim to provide this evidence through the comparison of a corpus of professionally-written research articles in Dental Public Health and a learner corpus of CHP projects produced by students from the Faculty of Dentistry, in the form of Contrastive Interlanguage Analysis (CIA, Granger, 1996, 2015). CIA is an attempt to "discover the features of nativeness and non-nativeness of learner language by comparing it with native language" (Gilquin, 2000: p. 95). To avoid the comparative fallacy of considering L1/L2 data as directly comparable (Bley-Vroman, 1989), we consider both expert and learner corpora as *varieties* under the CIA^2 model (Granger, 2015), where reference language varieties may be compared against interlanguage varieties, either of which can be set according to dialectic or diatypic variables (in this case, research articles for Dental Public Health).

3.2 Corpora for investigation

3.2.1 Professional Dentistry Corpus – Community Dental Health

Our professional community dentistry corpus is a collection of recent scholarly written articles published in the domain-specific journal *Community Dental Health* between 2010 and 2012. The journal represents a wide selection of public health issues in dentistry that are not only highly relevant to the Faculty's CHP projects but also provide input for the ED course. The journal publishes four issues annually with ten research articles per issue. When building the corpus, we omitted editorials, news, reviews and commentary articles from our corpus, ensuring that only research reports were included. The journal has a suggested word limit of 3,000 words per article. Although there is no mention of specific language features in the journal's style guide, authors are recommended to be "consistent with clarity of communication" (c.f. journal's website, n.d.). Permission to use the data for this purpose was granted by the journal's editor. After cleaning of the data, the corpus was comprised of 364,480 word tokens across 156 research articles. This corpus was to serve as a benchmark reference regarding the language characteristics, stylistic features, academic conventions, and common features of stance presentation in community-focused dentistry writing, against which the novice data would be compared.

3.2.2 Learner Corpus of Dentistry Reports

The learner corpus is comprised of students' fifth-year dentistry CHP reports, which after cleaning, totalled 525,140 words across 133 texts written between 1984 and 2010 (approximately 6 texts are produced per year). While students have produced these reports since 1984, the ED training on CHPs only began in 2016 following the start of the new 6-year dental curriculum in 2012, and so this collection of reports are all taken from the pre-ED period. As the major assessed work of CHPs, these reports are produced in small groups of 6–8 students. The reports are accessible in electronic form to staff and the general public as licensed by the university's library. Each text received at least a passing grade from a disciplinary tutor, with some awarded a distinction. The handbook for the CHP suggests that CHP projects must be relevant to Hong Kong, of current interest, manageable in terms of time and resources, of interest to the whole group of writers, and from within the broad field of dental public health. The handbook also advises dentistry students to structure their CHP reports beginning with an abstract, followed by an introduction including aims and objectives, materials and methods, results, discussion, conclusion and recommendations sections. However, the handbook offers no details specific to the language used in writing the reports. Since the first launch of the CHPs in 1984, student groups have been allocated 'project advisors' to oversee their work. These are not language teachers, but disciplinary tutors. Historically these tutors have provided very little (if any) feedback on language issues. Rather, the language-specific provision from the ED course is intended to meet the needs of students in the absence of language-specific feedback from disciplinary tutors. The novice texts are therefore indicative of the standard of the CHP reports as written before the introduction of the ED course.

Despite having the smaller number of texts (Table 3.1), the dentistry learner corpus is the larger corpus in terms of overall word count, with an average text length almost double that of texts in the professional corpus. This is due to the word limit restrictions imposed by the journal *Community Dental Health*. We note that a potential issue in comparing these learner and professional corpora is that

Table 3.1 Corpus size (whole texts, excluding references and appendices)

Corpus	Texts	Words	Av. text length (words)
Dentistry learner corpus	133	525,140	3,948.42
Professional dentistry corpus	156	364,680	2,337.69

the former is composed of project reports while the latter is composed of research reports, which may raise questions about their comparability. However, the university's dental faculty used the *Community Dental Health* journal as the inspiration for the CHP report capstone assessment. Moreover, given the overall research focus of the CHPs, the identical structure of the novice/professional texts, and the focus of both corpora on a very narrow field (Dental Public Health within local communities), we feel these corpora are as comparable as possible under a CIA^2 framework involving novice and professional writing.

3.3 Analysis 1: Multidimensional analysis

We begin our analyses of these two corpora using exploratory factor analysis (EFA) to conduct a multidimensional analysis (MDA) of the language features of the professional corpus, so to identify the latent correlations of linguistic features specific to professional practice in Public Dental Health writing before comparing these with the learner corpus. We must state here that this analysis was conducted in SPSS prior to our later adoption of JASP for statistical work, and so the goodness-of-fit statistics reported here use alternative measures from those in Chapter 2. Again, the freely available *Multidimensional Analysis Tagger* (MAT, Nini, 2015a) was used as the preferred software for isolation and annotation of linguistic features in the corpus. 31 features from the MAT analysis remained in the final EFA after removing features with low communality values (indicating they would struggle to load onto any factor) and/or for lack of frequency in the data. For the EFA, the method of extraction used was that of maximum likelihood, with rotation again performed using the oblimin rotation (implying the factors produced may be correlated) with Kaiser normalisation, which was completed in 26 iterations.

A total of five dimensions were derived from the EFA, with minimum factor loadings of .400 for inclusion within a given dimension, with these five factors responsible for 50.01% of the total variance explained (Table 3.2). The model's Kaiser-Meyer-Olkin measure of sampling adequacy was .725 (χ^2;= 2,082.72). The Kaiser-Meyer-Olkin measure of sampling adequacy is a statistic that indicates the proportion of variance in our variables that might be caused by underlying factors, with higher numbers indicating that the EFA is appropriate for our data. The EFA also produced a significant Bartlett's test of sphericity (d.f. = 465, $p < .001$), suggesting that the proportion of variance in the corpus data will likely be caused by the underlying factors the EFA would generate, which further ensures the validity of the EFA procedure.

Table 3.2 Results of MDA from the professional corpus

Feature	Dimension 1	Dimension 2	Dimension 3	Dimension 4	Dimension 5
Past tense verbs	.992				
Present tense verbs	−.506				
Nouns (not nominalisations or gerunds)		−.904			
Nominalisations		.553			
Possibility modals		.412			
Verbs in base form		.497	.692		
Infinitives		.472	.690		
Adjectives			−.471		
Predictive modals			.418		
Total prepositional phrases				−.642	
Determiners				−.521	
Verbs with past participle				−.436	
First person pronouns				.419	
Second person pronouns					.695
Quantifier pronouns					.672
Third person pronouns					.460
Preposition or subordinate conjunction					.417

One point of concern was that Dimension 1 is only categorised by two linguistic features (past tense verbs vs. present tense verbs). However, other trial iterations of the EFA[16] also had these two features together as characteristic of a single dimension without other additional features. In addition, the sufficiently high loading of past tense verbs (and concomitant high negative loading of present tense verbs) leaves us confident that these two features alone are therefore constitutive of a dimension in their own right. As with the EFA in Chapter 2, the fifth factor isolated from the EFA did not have any negative features, but as the function derived appears to be a binary variable (animacy), we have kept this factor labelled as a 'dimension' rather than a 'function' in the manner of Chapter 2.

The features involved in each dimension were then converted into a single unified z-score for each dimension, per file. These z-scores were then computed

16. That is, with certain low communality features not removed, or with the EFA involving four/five fixed dimensions rather than based on eigenvalue

for the same features in the learner corpus, allowing us to directly compare the significance of any variation of these features across the professional and learner corpora (Table 3.3).

To determine whether there was significant variation in the dimension scores across the professional and learner corpora, a multivariate analysis of variance (MANOVA) was performed on the z-scores across the five dimensions (alpha = .01). The results suggest significant variance along the five dimensions across the two corpora ($F (1, 283) = 73.70$, $p < .001$, partial $ETA^2 = .566$, Wilk's lambda = .434). Post-hoc test (Bonferroni) scores for Dimension 1 ($F (1, 287) = 57.63$, $p < .001$, partial $ETA^2 = .167$), Dimension 2 ($F (1, 287) = 37.27$, $p < .001$, partial $ETA^2 = .115$), Dimension 3 ($F (1, 287) = 121.22$, $p < .001$, partial $ETA^2 = .297$), Dimension 4 ($F (1, 287) = 133.77$, $p < .001$, partial $ETA^2 = .318$) and Dimension 5 ($F (1, 287) = 77.02$, $p < .001$, partial $ETA^2 = .212$) suggest each individual dimension was responsible for significant variation across the two corpora, with an effect size order of Dimensions 4, 3, 5, 1 and 2 respectively. Given this variation, we now characterise each dimension in more detail with reference to the statistics for each corpus and supported by examples from corpus texts.

3.3.1 Dimension 1 – Narrative vs. Informative

We have labelled the two poles of Dimension 1 (+) **Narrative vs. (–) Informative**, with past tense verbs as positive features along this dimension, and present tense verbs as negative features. According to Biber's Dimension 1 (1988), the use of past tense verbs is a narrative feature, unlike present tense verbs which serve an informative function. The dentistry students' research reports generally utilize a variety of past tense verbs as a form of 'story-telling' when offering their interpretation of their findings, or as a 'personal event' when relaying these findings to the general community – a finding also seen in the extensive use of first-person pronouns (see Dimension 4). An additional function specific to novice texts was the tendency to restate the findings from their results (usually in the form of tables) in prose in the discussion section:

> Findings from our survey indicated that median income levels amongst dentists were higher than what was reported in a 2000 survey conducted in Hong Kong. In our survey, the specialists reported to earning a higher monthly income compared with GDPs. It has been reported that dental postgraduates are the highest income earners of all graduates from the University of Hong Kong [27]. Specialists in our survey were as likely to feel that they made back their financial investment as did the GDPs, and that their income met with their expectation.

Table 3.3 Comparison of derived dimensions across professional and learner corpora

Z-scores	Learner	Professional
	(z-score, norm. freq. per 1000 tokens)	**(z-score, norm. freq. per 1000 tokens)**
Dimension 1	0.18	−0.15
Past tense verbs	.58 (4.14)	−.49 (3.07)
Present tense verbs	−.21 (1.82)	.18 (2.12)
Dimension 2	0.16	−0.42
Nouns (not nominalisations or gerunds)	−.64 (28.98)	−.75 (33.72)
Nominalisations	−.07 (4.49)	−.06 (4.30)
Possibility modals	.33 (0.45)	−.28 (0.33)
Verbs in base form	.61 (2.50)	−.52 (1.67)
Infinitives	.58 (1.36)	−.49 (0.92)
Dimension 3	0.36	−0.31
Verbs in base form	.61 (2.50)	−.52 (1.67)
Infinitives	.58 (1.36)	−.49 (0.92)
Adjectives	−.32 (8.56)	.27 (9.50)
Predictive modals	.59 (0.27)	−.51 (0.08)
Dimension 4	0.38	−0.32
Total prepositional phrases	.09 (11.80)	−.08 (11.69)
Determiners	.59 (8.30)	−.50 (6.50)
Verbs with past participle	.24 (2.58)	−.21 (3.30)
First-person pronouns	.60 (0.60)	−.51 (0.16)
Dimension 5	0.33	−0.28
Second-person pronouns	.06 (0.38)	−.05 (0.02)
Quantifier pronouns	.20 (0.10)	−.17 (0.004)
Third-person pronouns	.74 (1.19)	−.63 (0.42)
Preposition or subordinate conjunction	.34 (1.06)	−.29 (0.87)

Professional writers use a greater frequency of present tense verbs, communicating the current relevance of their research to readers who are already part of their professional community. They do so to categorize their research data, give their stance on the findings, and to communicate these findings as facts:

> Our finding is in line with the notion that dietary habits, pervading many aspects of people's daily lives, are hard to change, while brushing habits are more circumscribed and thus more ready to be modified (Rollnick et al., 1999). Furthermore, toothbrushing may appear to be a direct and effective solution to eradicate 'tooth worms' from the mouth, while controlling sweets as a way of 'starving' the tooth worms may be regarded as indirect and less appealing.

3.3.2 Dimension 2 – Persuasive vs. Objective

We have labelled the two poles of Dimension 2 (+) **Persuasive vs. (–) Objective**. This dimension is characterized by the occurrence of possibility modals, infinitives, and associated base form verbs on the positive cline, with nominalisations and nouns appearing on the negative cline of this dimension. Possibility modals are used by dentistry students in their research reports when hedging their findings, expressing their tentative novice perspectives about the findings of their projects rather than stating them as truths. These are also used when making recommendations (also requiring infinitives and base forms), which are significantly more frequent in the learner research reports than in the professionally-written research reports. The novice writers are interested in drawing clear links between their results and their impact on the local community, but do so cautiously via the use of hedges.

> The relation between patient's knowledge and previous treatment according to different age groups respectively seems to indicate that people in middle age group tend to know more. This may be explained by, firstly, every one's knowledge is perhaps directly related to their personal experience. Therefore, the more previous treatments they have, the more knowledge they might get. Secondly, in 1960, water fluoridation was introduced in Hong Kong and the middle age group may be the last group of people without any water fluoridation in their childhood. Consequently, they are likely more prone to caries and may have experienced more restorative treatment.

In the professional reports, nouns are much more frequently used, a practice associated with conveying dense information and allowing researchers to present their findings in a specific, accurate, and 'objective' manner.

> An overwhelming majority of the comments raised during the forums and contained in the written submissions could be classified as anti-fluoridationist. Their arguments are by no means unique and are common themes expressed by anti-fluoridationists nationally and internationally (Forum on Fluoridation, 2002; Armfield, 2007). As was similar to the Irish Forum on Fluoridation (2002), the true value of these submissions and comments was in bringing to light the range of concerns that needed to be addressed during the community education program. The Council in making the decision to fluoridate felt that the concerns and issues raised in the written submissions received from those opposed to the introduction of fluoridation had been adequately addressed by the community education program and responses provided by the NSW Health Department.

3.3.3 Dimension 3 – Tentative vs. Authoritative

We have labelled the two poles of Dimension 3 (+) **Tentative vs. (–) Authoritative.** On the positive cline, Dimension 3 is characterized by the co-occurrence of predictive modals and infinitives (with associated base forms). Novice writers tend to pose more possibilities arising from the findings, and as noted for Dimension 2, make many tentative recommendations based on their findings:

> As most of the pregnant women need regular medical check-up, it will be a good chance to provide dental health education during this period. However 58 (47.9%) of House Officers believed that calcium would be lost from teeth during pregnancy, this misconception needs to be corrected. On the whole, the majority of the interviewees were able to identify common dental diseases, and most of them would manage this by referring patients to dentists for appropriate treatment.

However, evaluative adjectives are commonly used as a persuasive tool to disseminate knowledge in professional writing, with authors describing the qualities of their findings in specific detail rather than taking a suggestive stance:

> Self-rated oral health has been found as an important determinant of the utilisation of dental services. Further- more, it is interesting that while in bivariate analysis better self-rated oral health was associated with greater likelihood of dental utilisation, in multivariate analysis the relationship was inversed. After controlling for the remaining variables of the model, better self-rated oral health is associated with lower dental utilisation. This highlights the important role of socio-economic variables which mediate critically the effect between perceived oral health and dental services utilisation. Socio-economic variables (namely income and education), even in the presence of insurance, are significant determinants of dental utilisation, a finding previously reported. (Millar and Locker, 1999)

3.3.4 Dimension 4 – Active vs. Passive

We have labelled the two poles of Dimension 4 (+) **Active vs. (–) Passive.** On the positive end of this dimension are first-person pronouns, with verbs in past participle on the negative side. First-person pronouns are frequently used by the novice writers, demonstrating a strong element of personal intrusion on the part of the students themselves into their texts. This provides an immediate human presence, again leaving the reader with the impression that the students are telling their research 'story'.

> In our questionnaire, there was a section which welcomed the visitors to express any comments towards this homepage. We received positive comments like, "this homepage is very interesting", "background music is very nice" and "the comics are good". We also obtained some negative comments, for example: "this homepage is too boring", "the pictures are ugly" and "background music is annoying".

The limited use of first-person pronouns in professional writing suggests a more passive and indirect approach, and the increased use of the passive voice (evidenced by verbs in the past participle) allows researchers to emphasise what was done rather than who was doing it.

> It has been documented that a high prevalence of untreated dental caries was associated with poor perceived oral health (Pattussi et al 2007). Secondly, oral health promoting behaviours such as routine dental attendance and diligent oral self-care was shown to be associated with inverse gradients in oral impacts (Sanders and Spencer, 2006). It was evident from the results of this study that oral health promoting behaviours such as frequency of tooth brushing and use of dental services has been increasing significantly with the increase in social status. Thus it is possible that these differences have been contributing to the observed social gradients in perceived oral health outcomes.

3.3.5 Dimension 5 – Animate vs. Inanimate

We have labelled the two poles of Dimension 5 (+) **Animate vs. (–) Inanimate**. The use of second- and third-person pronouns as a positive feature of this dimension is seen frequently in student writing when relaying interview or questionnaire data directed at research participants, often including the questions themselves in the reported results, for example "we asked the patient 'are you feeling comfortable?'". They also use these forms when describing their patients, maintaining a human, animate type of reference in keeping with the narrative style of their research reports:.

> Only very few of the subjects did not have their own toothbrush (Figure 7). About 90% of the subjects brushed their teeth with fluoridated dentifrice, but the rest did not know which brand they were using (Figure 8). All subjects employed toothbrushing as their daily means of cleaning teeth. In addition, some rinsed their mouth after meals while only a few of them use toothpicks and floss (Figure 9). The participants reported that they brushed their teeth more frequently than non-participants (Figure 10). More than half of the participants claimed that they brushed their teeth twice daily, and in fact, one third claimed that they brushed 3 times daily.

The lack of these features in the professional research reports reflects the objective, if dehumanising nature of professionally written texts within this genre, with professional writers referring to patients nominally, or in the form of numerical conversions:.

> Evaluation of 65,236 files of newborns in 12 hospitals of Yazd province over a four-year period between 2003 and 2006 revealed cleft defects in 56 newborns. The present study showed that cleft lip and palate was seen in 0.86/1000 births or in other words, 1/1165 births. In populations of Poland (Antoszewski et al. 1997), Germany (Hruskova et al. 1998), U.S.A (Tolarova et al. 1998) and Korea (Kim et al. 2002), the prevalence of cleft lip and palate was 1.85, 2, 1.3 and 1.81 per 1,000, respectively

3.4 Analysis 2: Making claims personal: Hedging, boosting and self-mention[17]

The findings above regarding Dimensions 2 and 3 suggest a persuasive, authoritative approach to writing in professionally-written texts as contrasted with that of more tentative novice writing. We now turn our attention to the lexical features of these continua across the two corpora, with reference to particular sections found in these reports (e.g. introduction, results, discussion) where authors employ persuasive or tentative language. Here, we focus on the linguistic forms used for the functions of hedging, boosting, and self-mention, each a key component of the writers' presentation of stance (Hyland, 2005). Hedges, or "words or phrases whose job it is to make things fuzzier" (Lakoff, 1972: 195), allow the writer to express his or her lack of commitment to the certainty of the information given, while boosters allow writers to express their confidence about the validity of a proposition (Holmes, 1988; Hu & Cao, 2015; Hyland, 2005). Hedges and boosters are not only crucial in academic discourse but are also seen as a central rhetorical device in science discourse to gain communal adherence to knowledge claims and build interpersonal solidarity with readers (Hyland, 1999; Lancaster, 2016). Although self-mentions project writers' explicit presence and effectuate affective persuasion, they are not highly expected in scientific writing, which may privilege cloaking authors as humble servants to scientific methods (Biber, 2006b; Hyland, 2005).

The data were converted for annotation with the freely available *UAM Corpustool* (Version 3.3., O'Donnell, 2008)[18]. UAM allows for both manual and automatic annotation using regular expressions to bring up all instances of a given word or phrase, which can then be annotated simultaneously. The choice of hedges, boosters and self-mention to be investigated in this study matches a

17. Text, tables, and charts of this analysis have been reproduced from Crosthwaite, Chung & Jiang (2017), in *English for Specific Purposes*. We express our gratitude to Elsevier for permitting us to reproduce this analysis for this volume under license.

18. http://www.corpustool.com/

general, non-disciplinary list of these features presented in an appendix within Hyland (2000), rather than compiling a list of dentistry stance features from the professional corpus before comparing their occurrence with the learner data. Doing the latter would firstly risk committing the comparative fallacy, and secondly risk omitting any non-discipline-specific devices used in the learner data from the analysis. Each annotated occurrence of these items was then double-checked by the authors and a research assistant of near-native English proficiency along a 9-word context concordance line to ensure that each occurrence fulfilled its stated metadiscoursal function (e.g. if a booster such as 'clear' was preceded with 'not', this would be a hedging rather than a boosting device). Having bilingual English/Cantonese speakers check the annotation follows the suggestion of Dagneaux, Denness and Granger (1998) in that "efficiency is increased" if the annotator has both a high knowledge of English grammar and the L1 mother tongue of the interlanguage variety to be analysed (p. 165). For analysis of cross-corpus frequencies, due to differences in corpus sizes, the raw frequencies of the annotated items were converted into normalised frequencies per 1,000 words in UAM. The frequencies for each file in the corpus were then exported to an Excel document then converted into an SPSS-ready file (v.20) for statistical analysis.

For analysis of wordings, we generated wordlists from both learner and professional corpora that include the raw frequency of the annotated lexical items in UAM, before entering this data into the *Log-likelihood Calculator* (Rayson, 2016) to determine the keyness of the individual items. Significance values of $p < 0.001$ are given for *LL* values of greater than 10.83, and significance values of $p < 0.0001$ are given for *LL* values of greater than 15.13. Effect sizes for log-likelihood are also provided, following the Bayes Information Criterion (BIC) measure (Wilson, 2013). Table 3.4 shows the annotated features (hedges, boosters, self-mention) of the two corpora by section, as well as the word counts and average section lengths of each respective section.

Despite being one of the shortest sections in each corpus, the limitations sections found in the professional dentistry corpus are three times longer than those found in the learner dentistry corpus. As the limitations section is a section where hedging the findings of the study would be most likely to occur, it is apparent that the novice writers do not tend to focus on the limitations of their studies. This could be because students are aware their research reports are assessed, and they wish to emphasize the importance of their research findings over any limitations of their study so as to impress the examiners. The second point of interest is that the recommendations sections of texts in the learner corpus are almost three times longer than those of the professional corpus. Novice writers appear to devote more space to emphasising any links between their research findings and their potential impact on Hong Kong community dental health.

Table 3.4 Annotated features and corpus size (by section)

Corpus	Words	Av. section length	Annotated items
Dentistry learner corpus			
Abstract	33,929	255.1	H = 379, B = 262, SM = 105
Introduction	71,306	536.13	H = 1213, B = 514, SM = 358
Method	99,294	746.57	H = 677, B = 248, SM = 777
Results	157,641	1,185.27	H = 2439, B = 1191, SM = 376
Discussion	130,717	982.83	H = 3288, B = 1371, SM = 1349
Limitations	3,013	22.65	H = 192, B = 11, SM = 77
Conclusion	16,383	123.18	H = 269, B = 141, SM = 131
Recommendations	12,857	96.66	H = 200, B = 75, SM = 152
Professional dentistry corpus			
Abstract	29,823	224.23	H = 252, B = 131, SM = 105
Introduction	51,422	386.63	H = 714, B = 318, SM = 29
Method	80,721	606.92	H = 504, B = 180, SM = 161
Results	74,161	557.6	H = 759, B = 585, SM = 55
Discussion	103,543	778.51	H = 2061, B = 847, SM = 324
Limitations	8,023	60.32	H = 69, B = 55, SM = 54
Conclusion	11,356	85.38	H = 214, B = 115, SM = 28
Recommendations	5,631	42.33	H = 88, B = 35, SM = 12

(H = Hedges, B = Boosters, SM = Self-mention)

Table 3.5 shows the cross-corpora distribution of stance devices. To correct for multiple testing (avoiding 'data dredging/fishing', where multiple tests can lead to false significance, see Young & Karr, 2011), an alpha value of 0.0125 (for 4 tests)[19] was used to ascertain the significance of the Mann-Whitney U comparison, with Holm-Bonferroni correction on the *p* values. As non-parametric statistics were performed, the median/absolute deviations are reported instead of the mean / standard deviations.

There are significant differences in the frequencies of hedges, boosters and self-mentions between the learner and professional corpora. In each case, the learner data contains a significantly higher frequency of each type of metadiscourse over that of professionally-written reports, with medium effect sizes noted for both hedges and boosters and large effect sizes noted for self-mentions. We now turn to the use of these features by section of the report.

19. The original version of this analysis (Crosthwaite, Cheung & Jiang, 2017) also looked at attitude markers. As the findings for hedges, boosters and self-mention were significant at the lower alpha value in that paper (four tests = 0.0125), we have retained the original statistics from that analysis rather than re-do them here with higher (less conservative) alpha values for three metadiscourse features.

Table 3.5 Cross-corpora comparison of stance markers.

Feature	Median/AD per 1,000 words	Mann-Whitney	Effect size (Pearson's r)
Hedges	Dent. Learner, M = 9.86, AD = 2.38 Dent. Prof., M = 6.85, AD = 1.91	U = 4,907, t = −7.72, $p < .001$	$r = -0.454$
Boosters	Dent. Learner, M = 4.44, AD = 1.08 Dent. Prof. M = 3.35, AD = 0.88	U = 6,057, t = −6.09, $p < .001$	$r = -0.359$
Self-Mention	Dent. Learner, M = 4.24, AD = 2.17 Dent. Prof. M = 0.67, AD = 0.45	U = 2,312, t = −11.38, $p < .001$	$r = -0.670$

Pearson R Effect size interpretation, .10 = 'small', .30 = 'medium', .50 = 'large', .70 = 'very large', Cohen (1988).

3.4.1 Hedging

The learner dentistry reports contain a significantly higher frequency of linguistic devices used for hedging compared to that of the professional dentistry reports. Using Mann-Whitney U analyses to compare both corpora by section, we found that the learner CHP writers were significantly more likely to use hedging devices in all sections bar the recommendations section (where the professional writers were more likely to use hedging). (See Figure 3.1.) Small effect sizes (Pearson's r) are found for the abstract, limitations, and conclusion sections, medium effect sizes for the method and results sections, and large effect sizes for the introduction – when hedging the claims of others – and discussion sections – when hedging their own claims. An investigation of the lexical items used as hedging devices between the two corpora provides a potential explanation (Table 3.6).

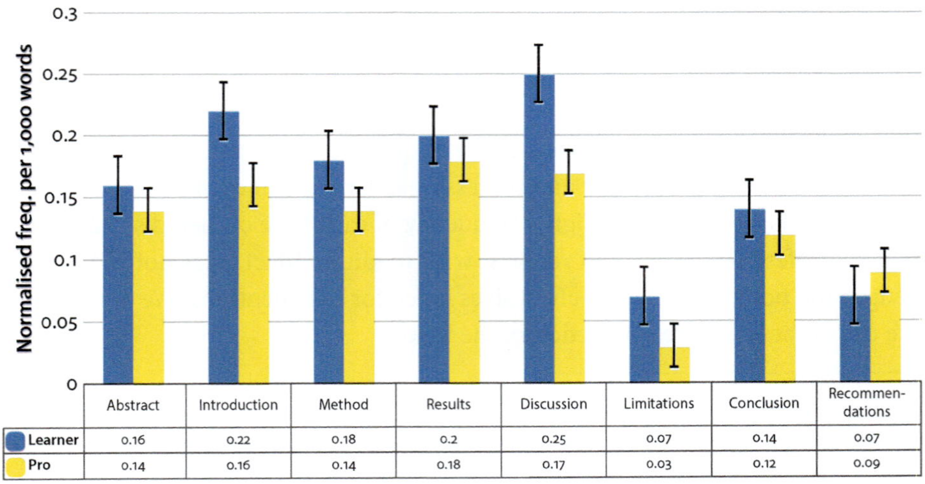

Figure 3.1 Use of hedging devices in learner and professional reports (by section)

Table 3.6 Lexical items used as hedges (Minimum LL 15.13, $p < .0001$)

Word	Freq. DL	Freq. PRO	Specific to DL vs. PRO	Log likelihood	Effect size (BIC)
about	720	93	DL	381.24	367.43
would	1,338	345	DL	368.90	355.08
claimed	323	30	DL	205.15	191.34
quite	220	20	DL	141.14	127.33
could	909	398	DL	82.63	91.91
felt	210	45	DL	72.63	84.73
mainly	259	47	DL	105.72	68.82
usually	218	52	DL	66.53	52.72
generally	191	62	DL	36.35	22.54
might	361	172	DL	24.23	10.42
probably	111	37	DL	20.07	6.26
sometimes	63	16	DL	17.73	3.92
maybe	38	6	DL	17.44	3.63
indicating	0	78	PRO	132.87	119.06
estimated	1	69	PRO	50.94	94.36
estimates	1	53	PRO	81.44	67.63
estimate	23	61	PRO	30.88	17.07
often	132	175	PRO	25.42	11.61
assumed	11	38	PRO	24.78	10.97
indicates	32	63	PRO	21.53	7.72
suggests	27	56	PRO	20.72	6.91

BIC effect size: 0–2: low effect, 2–6: positive evidence against the null hypothesis (H0), 6–10: strong evidence against H0, > 10: very strong evidence against H0 (Wilson, 2013)

There are significant (i.e. $p < .0001$) differences in the wordings used for hedging between learner and professional texts. Professional writers appear to use the lemmas 'indicate', 'estimate' and 'suggests' frequently, with these lemmas most often used to hedge the author's own claims:

> Although the cost-effectiveness of preventive measures may vary according to the size of the community, the overall results indicating a favourable trend in the assessment of dental caries prevention programme from a societal perspective … This study also estimates the likely impact on DMFT indicators of excluding the 15% of children with lower capacity to understand a simple explanation …
>
> Thus overall there has been an increase in the ratio of the caries prevalence for the most deprived fifth to the middle fifth across the two survey years from 1.18 (53.8%/45.5%) in 2004–05 to 1.24 (52.4%/42.1%) in 2008–09. This suggests that there has been a widening of the inequalities gap in Wales …

Learner writers, on the other hand, hedge the claims of others with 'claimed' and 'felt', while hedging the reporting of behaviour with 'usually', 'generally', 'sometimes', and explicitly expressing uncertainty with 'might', 'probably', or 'maybe'. They are also more likely to express conditional epistemology via modals such as 'could' and 'would', hedge numerical information with 'about', and evaluate attributive information with 'quite'.

> Over three-quarters (83%, 399) of the study participants claimed that they experienced an oral health problems in the past …
>
> Patients can usually come up with a multitude of excuses to avoid or escape from dental treatment, such as a lack of time or money …
>
> This in part may relate to the effects of drug abuse on caries experience or is maybe just a reflection of the underlying social background of the group …
>
> About one third of the people with SSc in this study showed a XI score equal to or more than 30. This could mean that SSc has a larger effect on some Chinese people with SSc in Hong Kong or more severe self-reported symptoms of dry mouth could be resulted from more severe scleroderma …
>
> Fifty-six point four percent of private dental practitioners preferred an item-based payment method and about 90% of them were willing to provide oral examinations and scaling for the proposed scheme …
>
> The participants were quite evenly distributed amongst the group according to relevant working experience, 41.4% of them had 5 years or less working experience while 31.7% of them had worked for more than 10 years …

Professional writers, while less frequently hedging both their and others' claims, tend also not to hedge with adverbs and modals, instead using specific verbs to convey uncertainty or to be careful about expressing any claim made in the text. There was no correlation found between the date of the learner reports and the use of hedging devices, implying that, as yet, there has been little impact of any English language training on the use of such devices, or that the conditions under which the texts are produced are encouraging the learner writers to frequently hedge their claims.

3.4.2 Boosting

The findings here suggest that professional writers use a significantly higher frequency of boosting devices in the introduction, results, discussion, and limitations sections. (See Figure 3.2.) This finding is apparently at odds with the finding shown in Table 3.5 that, across the entire text, learner writers tend to boost their claims more frequently than professional writers. Medium to large effect sizes are noted for the introduction, results, and discussion sections – particularly the discussion section,

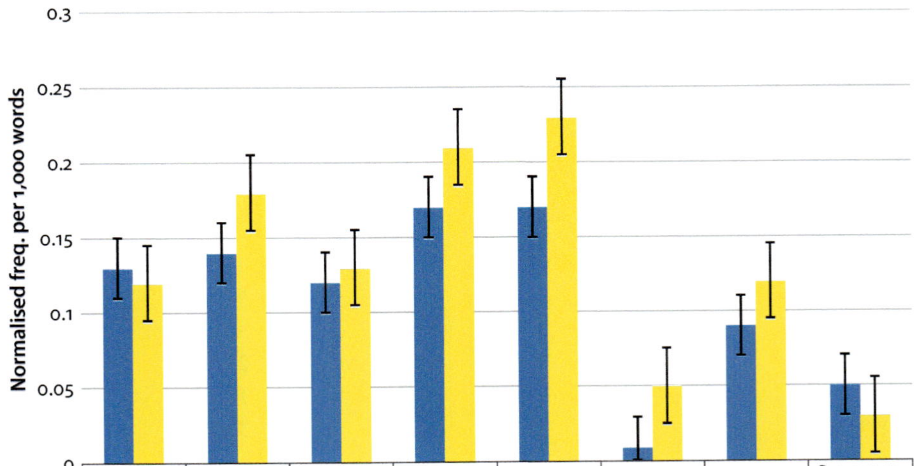

	Abstract	Introduction	Method	Results	Discussion	Limitations	Conclusion	Recommen-dations
Learner	0.13	0.14	0.12	0.17	0.17	0.009	0.09	0.05
Pro	0.12	0.18	0.13	0.21	0.23	0.05	0.12	0.03

Figure 3.2 Frequency of boosting devices used between learner and professional reports

where the professional writers are boosting their own claims based on their research findings. By way of explanation, the LL results (Table 3.7) for boosters show that the learner writers used certain boosters (e.g. 'found') with a very high frequency, yet this use is presumably concentrated in the few sections (abstract, recommendations) where the learners used more boosters than the professional writers.

Despite the finding at the section level that professional writers appear to boost claims more frequently than seen in learner writing, there are clear differences in the lexical items used between professional and learner writers in this regard. Professional writers tend to use variations of the verbs 'show' and 'demonstrate' when boosting their and others' claims, focusing on their findings rather than their or others' personal feelings or actions.

> Taken together, the results from across England Scotland and Wales <u>show</u> that the trend for reducing caries prevalence and severity continues in this age group in all three countries …
>
> The results obtained from this study <u>demonstrate</u> that periodontal disease among people over 75 years of age is more prevalent and more severe in the Puerto Rican population than in the overall US population, or among US Hispanics of similar age …

On the other hand, learner writers tend to consider their or others' thought processes via verbs such as 'thought', 'know', 'thinking', and 'believed', their or others'

Table 3.7 Lexical items used for boosting (Minimum LL 15.13, p < .0001)

Word	Freq. DL	Freq. PRO	Specific to DL or PRO	Log likelihood	Effect size (BIC)
thought	308	0	DL	342.65	328.84
found	1,120	628	DL	32.99	106.80
know	216	28	DL	114.10	100.29
think	96	0	DL	106.80	92.99
obvious	50	0	DL	55.62	41.81
clear	49	0	DL	54.51	40.70
believed	132	37	DL	32.24	18.13
find	125	37	DL	28.00	14.19
in fact	76	21	DL	18.97	5.16
never	138	55	DL	33.35	2.74
----------	-----------	------------	------------	----------	---------
shows	5	117	PRO	163.14	149.33
shown	149	207	PRO	34.37	20.56
showing	9	40	PRO	31.41	17.60
demonstrating	0	12	PRO	20.44	6.63
demonstrated	66	99	PRO	19.98	6.17
finding	0	10	PRO	17.03	3.22
establishing	0	9	PRO	15.33	1.52

actions via the use of 'find'/'found', and also point out 'apparent' truths via adjectives such as 'obvious' and 'clear' and via adverbs such as 'in fact' and 'never'.

> The majority of them (91/159) thought that they had no perceived dental problem and a small group of them (13/159) thought dental treatments cost too much …

> Since the proposed periodontal treatment needs of the study subjects are based on their CPI scores, it is not surprising to find that the treatment needs of the subjects in the above three studies were similar …

> From our survey findings, it is obvious that there is a need for dental health education programmes on dental trauma management to be delivered to the teacher trainees in Hong Kong …

3.4.3 Self-mentions

With the exception of the discussion and limitations sections, the learner dentistry reports contained a significantly higher number of self-mentions compared with those in professionally written texts (Figure 3.3). Learner writers frequently used the personal plural pronouns 'our', 'we', and 'us'. One potential reason for

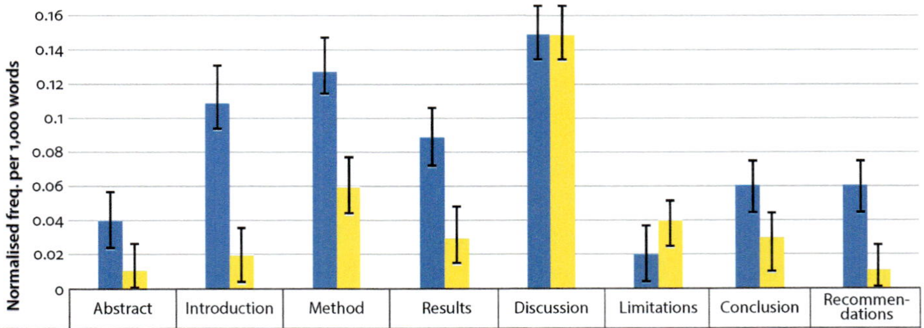

	Abstract	Introduction	Method	Results	Discussion	Limitations	Conclusion	Recommen-dations
Learner	0.04	0.11	0.13	0.09	0.15	0.02	0.06	0.06
Pro	0.01	0.02	0.06	0.03	0.15	0.04	0.03	0.01

Figure 3.3 Frequency of self-mention used between learner and professional reports by section

this is that the learner dentistry reports were all group projects, while some of the texts in the professional corpus may have been written by single authors. However, as both learner and professional texts have been anonymised, we are unaware of which papers were produced by single/multiple authors. The use of 'our' in the learner reports was mostly linked to mentions of the student 'group' (LL = 126.79, p < .001, BIC = 102.98), or various words related to the project itself, including 'project' (LL = 354.89, p < .001, BIC = 341.08). This stands in contrast to the use of 'our' in professional written texts, which tended to be used for mention of 'data' (LL = 18.74, p < .001, BIC = 4.92) in the discussion section.

> Our group chose a daily life approach to deliver the message of oral health awareness …
> Our project can provide information concerning the dental health status and treatment need of the children to the dentists serving the children there …
> There are reasons to believe that our data and the model have captured some of the social processes that were important for oral health development …

The five most frequent verbs following 'we' (except for the copula or modals) are 'found' (*n* = 100), 'decided' (*n* = 40), 'recommend' (*n* = 26), 'chose' (*n* = 25), and 'think' (*n* = 19), each of which convey a personal decision or suggestion made by the authors. Along with the increased use of 'us' compared to the professional texts, it is apparent from the data that learner writers make considerable use of pronominal self-mention in almost every section of their reports.

3.5 Narrative features of novice Dental Public Health writing: An NLP approach

The final analysis of this chapter involves the use of NLP software to confirm the findings of the MDA regarding Dimensions 1 (Narrative vs. Informative) and 5 (Animate vs. Inanimate). Here, we utilise the freely available *Ubiqu+Ity* (version 1.2), which is an online environment for corpus-based rhetorical analysis made available through the University of Wisconsin-Madison. This web-based software annotates text files for features present under the *Docuscope* dictionary (Kaufer & Butler 1996, 2000; Kaufer, Ishizaki, Butler & Collins 2004). We used Version 3.85[20] of the *Docuscope* dictionary as available in *Ubiqu+Ity*, annotating our text files across 170 rhetorical categories. We contacted the authors of the software for the complete list of these categories and their respective subcategories with examples, but they were unable to provide these. Analysis simply involved adding the files for each corpus into a .zip file and uploading this file to the *Ubiqu+Ity* front-end, where it is processed online before the software creates a .csv file with the statistics for each file in the corpus, which we then converted to an SPSS-ready file. The software comes with a viewer package to allow you to see a visual representation of each code, as shown in Figure 3.4. Here, one can see the coding for the *academic_specialised* feature in the document and as represented by the density of this coding across the document in the chart on the right. However, at present the software can only provide this visualisation per file rather than across the whole corpus.

The normalised frequencies of each feature were transformed into standardized z-scores, which allows for relative frequency differences across a wide range of features within the corpus to be less of a confounding factor when performing regression analysis. A binary logistic regression analysis was performed on the data with the learner corpus as the target for the regression and the professional corpus as the reference category. This ensured that we could determine which features were positive predictors of the learner data and which would necessarily be lacking in the professional data. This also left any negative predictors of the learner data as *de-facto* positive predictors of the professional data. The regression was performed using a stepwise procedure, using the Wald statistic as the condition for factors to remain in the model for each step.

The analysis (Table 3.8) resulted in seven of the rhetorical features annotated in *Ubiqu+Ity* being derived as significant predictors of the learner data, with five positive predictors and two negative predictors. The model had excellent predictive power (-2LL = 43.44, Nagelkerke R^2 = .950) and passed goodness-of-fit tests (Hosmer & Lemeshow χ^2 = 1.24, df = 8, sig = .996).

20. The next version, Version 3.91, contains 1878 categories, with 2426 categories in Version 4, the latest version – perhaps overkill for our needs!

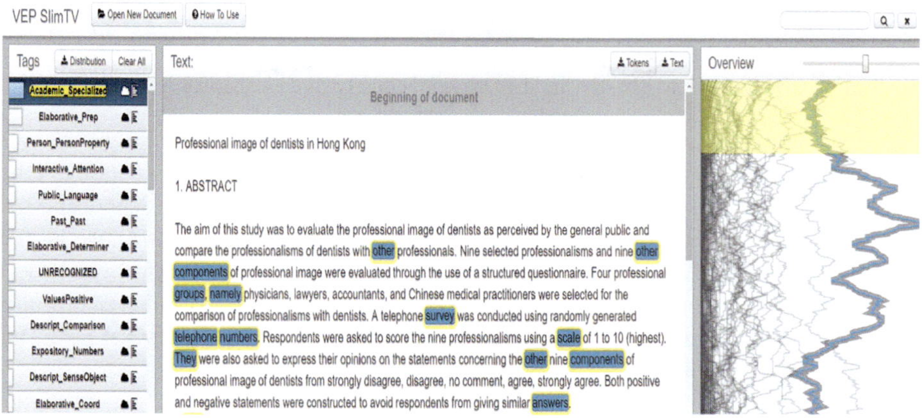

Figure 3.4 Text analysis visualisation in the *Ubiqu+Ity* environment

Two of the positive predictors of the learner data were found in the 'description' rhetorical group. The *sense_object* feature relates to specific objects involved in descriptions of places or areas, often provided as background information for the reader before shifting back to retelling the events in the foreground – a typical feature of narrative prose (Hopper & Thompson, 1980). In this example, the dentistry novice group is reporting the ideal layout of a dental practice reception:

> This [the reception] is the most important area in terms of patients' first impression of the practice. It conveys a feeling of warmth and concern to the patient in the design and decor. The number of seats in the area depends on the available space but the seats should be comfortable. Lighting should be adequate for reading but not too harsh as to create tension. Colours should be warm to provide a feeling of comfort and care. Magazines and umbrella stands may also be provided. If space allows, a small children's corner with toys and books can be included.

Table 3.8 Results of regression analysis for *Ubiqu+Ity* rhetorical features across corpora

Feature	Norm freq. DL	Norm freq. PRO	β	Sig.	(exp)β effect size
Citation (Advancing claims)	0.05	0.02	1.40	<.001	4.08
Description (Sense_object)	3.23	2.79	1.28	0.001	3.61
Past	3.18	2.09	2.33	<.001	10.32
Person (Property)	3.43	2.15	2.04	0.001	7.76
Description (Scene shifts)	0.51	0.32	1.59	0.007	4.94
----------	----------	----------	----------	----------	----------
Citation (Authority/Dates)	0.55	3.26	−5.30	<.001	0.005
Narrative (Time/Date)	0.08	0.17	−2.86	0.001	0.056

Regarding *scene shifts,* the novice writers displayed a tendency to report data collection activities in the form of a 'visit' or 'trip', with the research as a whole likened to that of a 'journey', as shown in this strongly narrative example:

> Our project planning commenced with a visit to Conghua in January 1988 by 2 student representatives together with teachers. At this visit, baseline data about the working environment and information about the Conghua health School and Liu Xi Primary School were gathered. After they returned to Hong Kong, we started our preparation, which included the design of the survey charting form and questionnaire, construction of exhibition boards, banners, posters, and even our uniforms! Before we set off for Conghua, we tested our survey methods at Lam Tim Siu Kwong Primary School under the supervision of Dr. Li.

Interestingly, under the 'narrative' rhetorical group, the only significant predictor of either corpus was that of *time and date*, and this was actually found in the professional corpus. In particular, the use of the phrase 'at the time of' featured heavily in a number of the professional texts, typically as a sentence opener:

> At the time of the original study, tooth wear on the labial and palatal surfaces of the upper central and lateral incisors was reported and assumed to have an erosive aetiology
>
> At the time of the examination, no attempt was made to distinguish between the different types of tooth wear, the index is descriptive.

Another significant predictor of the learner data was found for the *person_property* feature. *Person_property* relates to nouns that describe the property or occupation of people in terms of a standalone lexical item, adjectives modifying nouns, or adjectives themselves, and these features appear heavily in the learner texts in the descriptions of the communities where the projects were carried out.

> Oral health education was delivered to the adult and pre-school children in the Pillar Point Refugee Camp and the school children in the Yuen Long school run by International Social Service. Two sets of questionnaires were translated into Vietnamese from English with the help of the official interpreters in the Pillar Point Vietnamese Refugee Camp, one for the children (age 11–16, Appendix 1 and 2) and the other for the adults (age 20 +, Appendix 3 and 4). They were distributed to the Vietnamese refugees at the time of examination by the teachers in the school or interpreters in the camp. The adult group was interviewed by the interpreters individually while the children were divided into groups of seven guided by their teachers.

Another main example of *person_property* specific to the novice data (although not a narrative concern) is that of the relative overuse of the terms 'dentist' and 'patient', without using synonyms, substitutions or other referential means to describe these groups. These examples are suggestive of a more animate referential approach to novice writing than that seen in professional writing, further confirming the findings of the MDA for Dimension 5.

> Patient's satisfaction with dental care is a comparison between the patient's desires and perceptions of the dentist's duty. Such perceptions are mainly based on the dentist's general clinical performance, communication skills, and efficiency in running the clinic, rather than the dentist's technical work in which the patient cannot evaluate fully. [...] Patients who can appreciate the benefits of dental work bring less stress to dentists, which will increase the dentist's job motivation and satisfaction.

Regarding *past,* this involves almost all verbs in past tense, the heavy use of which is traditionally associated with narrative discourse (Biber, 1988). Finally, under the rhetorical function of *citation*, there appear to be two contrasting approaches between the learner and professional texts. The learner texts contained more frequent use of *advancing claims,* involving the construction 'X claims X' / 'X claimed X', referring directly to the author of the claim in subject position. These integral citations place prominence on the messenger (Swales, 1990). In the professional texts, authors tended to use non-integral citations in order to avoid specific mention of the author, focusing instead of the claim.

Dental caries remains the most significant dental public health problem in the UK and concerns have been expressed over the potentially rising prevalence of erosion (Office of National Statistics, 2003; Pitts et al., 2007). Obesity, especially in children, is increasing dramatically across the country (Jackson-Leach and Lobstein, 2006) and is associated with an increased risk of type 2 diabetes in the young (Drake et al., 2002).

The distribution of integral/non-integral citations between L2 and professional writers shown in these results is similar to that of other studies (e.g. Ädel & Garretson, 2006; Swales, 2014; Lee, Hitchcock & Casal, 2018) and is likely due to previous instruction (Swales, 2014).

3.6 Chapter summary

This chapter has presented three comparative, contrastive analyses of learner and professionally-written Dental Public Health research reports. Each analysis has shown a range of differences between novice and professional writing for this genre, indicative of the degree of membership to which each writer group resides in a situated model (Lave & Wenger, 1991). Each analysis is therefore significant food for thought for ESAP professionals wishing to enculturate novice writers into the rhetorical practices of the target profession. From the MDA analysis, five specific dimensions of linguistic features were derived from the EFA for the professional corpus. These were *narrative vs. informative, persuasive vs. objective, tentative vs. authoritative, active vs. passive* and *animate vs. inanimate.* The relative frequencies of these linguistic features were significantly different for each dimension across professional and learner writing. Namely, learner writing demonstrated a tendency for past tense over present tense verbs as well as first, second- and third-person pronouns as characteristic of a 'story-telling' function of novice reports. This tendency appeared alongside increased use of possibility modals (for hedging), predictive modals (for suggestions) and infinitives (to make recommendations). These findings allow us to summarise novice writing as narrative, overtly persuasive, overly tentative, primarily 'active' in argument structure and featuring more animate descriptions of entities than found in professional writing. Professional writers eschewed these linguistic features for devices resulting in more informative, objective, authoritative, and passive writing.

The results of the second analysis have again demonstrated significant differences between the two writer groups as evidenced in the varying frequencies of hedging, boosting and self-mention used, and the lexical items used to realise them. Variation is exhibited across whole texts and between individual sections of texts. Learner writers are shown to very frequently hedge and boost their claims, appearing simultaneously cautious and confident when considering certain claims made by others or by themselves, and are likely to frequently self-insert. Professional writers tend to use a narrower set of hedging and boosting verbs for these functions, unlike the wider range of adverbs and adjectives seen in the learner reports. It should be said that learner writers of these dentistry reports *are* able to hedge and boost the claims of others and their own claims within each relevant section of their reports, albeit doing so using a wider range of devices than those seen in professional texts.

For the final, automated analysis, the findings have confirmed those of the MDA regarding Dimensions 1 and 5. Learner texts were found to be more likely to contain a range of rhetorical features typically associated with narratives, and were more likely to refer to animate referents in their writing. As with almost any closed-source automated NLP software, there are likely to be a number of analyses that are unusable due to false-positives in the data, and this was certainly the case with *Ubiqu+Ity*. For example, *Ubiqu+Ity*'s analysis of *motions* under its *description* rhetorical group (a point of interest in determining narrative style) often results in false positives when considering the topic of the report. The document with the highest frequency of *motions* in the learner corpus was a study into how people with cerebral palsy coped with brushing, featuring both complex descriptions of the medical condition:

> Ataxic type – Ataxic means "shaking" and is uncommon nowadays (Howle, 2002). People with ataxia cannot walk steadily. They have poor balance in body movement and eye-hand coordination. Tremor may be present as well [...] Hemiplegia affects one side of the body only. Mobility is usually normal on one side while the other side limps or drags during walking or running.

This passage cannot be taken as evidence of a 'narrative' style to the learner writing – rather, this appears to be a valid description of the condition, similar to what would be present in the professional texts.

Our findings for both the learner and professionally written texts are in line with Gross and Chesley's (2012) suggestion that experts reduce the frequency of hedges (and presumably also boosters) used in order to support perceived objectivity, and Aull and Lancaster's (2014) finding that developing academic writers tend to use a high frequency of both hedges and boosters, albeit not always appropriately. In terms of implications of these findings for pedagogy, ESAP tutors need to devote time and space within the curriculum for explicit instruction on how present tense reporting verbs can be used purposefully to express stance on research findings (as seen for professional writing in Williams, 1996), how nouns and nominalisations can be used to present research findings in an accurate and objective manner (see also Jiang & Hyland, 2016), and how the tone of novice writing can be made more authoritative via the acquisition and use of discipline-appropriate evaluative adjectives (e.g. Swales & Burke, 2003). We suggest that ESAP teachers of dentistry discipline-specific writing would "best benefit from a process of further sensitising learners to the discursive norms of the research genre and rhetorical expectations of writing in the disciplines, beginning by narrowing the range of expressions used for hedging and boosting to those preferred in the professionally-written research reports investigated in the present study" (Crosthwaite, Cheung & Jiang, 2017: p. 119).

So, how to go about this process? Well, this is where we suggest placing the technology we have used to generate these findings firmly in the hands of those who need it the most – the ESAP students (as well as their tutors). Allowing students to query their own written work using integrated platforms such as *Ubiqu+Ity* could be a valuable experience, as the advantages afforded by the rapid automated analysis of thousands of rhetorical features across learner texts cannot be understated. Such results could serve as valuable ammunition for convincing students of the need to be aware of the importance and appropriacy of rhetorical features in their disciplinary writing. In particular, the highly visual nature of the output generated by such tools can serve to have an immediate effect on novice writers, even if they do not entirely understand the linguistic concepts behind them. However, this is likely too broad an approach for many. Rather, raising awareness of the issues raised in this chapter through targeted, guided student engagement with professional disciplinary corpora may be crucial in allowing students to discover and understand the rhetorical practices of professional writers. In addition, by including comparable learner corpora into the mix, student engagement with corpus data can and should lead students to discover and understand how their own writing is positioned in relation to that of the discipline of which they are to eventually become participating members. The pedagogical realisation, results and evaluation of our attempts in this area are described for the reader in Section 2 of this volume.

CHAPTER 4

Understanding disciplinary vs. non-disciplinary terminology

Insights from the dentistry case report genre

4.1 Introduction

This chapter marks a change in approach from the broad MDA-type analyses seen in Chapters 2 and 3 to focus more on disciplinary vocabulary within the case report genre of dentistry writing. Alongside experimental research articles, case reports are one of the crucial genres novice undergraduate dentists are frequently exposed to and are required to produce during their studies. However, unlike experimental research articles, which are likely to be written once a dentist has already been practicing for some time, novice dentists will be expected to produce some form of case reports almost immediately upon starting their clinical practice. Disciplinary tutors place great emphasis on the case report as a site for communicating the complexities involved in patient care, from initial diagnosis to provision of dental treatment, as well as dentist-patient interaction before and after dental procedures. Each step in this process has a potential impact on future clinical decisions regarding treatment. It is therefore highly important for dentistry students to internalise the language features of case reports so as to be able to understand the day-to-day work of a practicing dentist, and to be able to share their experiences with the profession once they have conducted their first clinical procedures.

In the previous three-year curriculum at the university, oral tasks on case reports were designed to develop first-year dentistry students' ability to evaluate a patient's treatment choices and to present clinical findings and treatment options to a mock patient in an appropriate way, before eventually disseminating this procedure in the form of a case report. Via a series of pair and group tasks, students were to understand the basic components of a case study (i.e. case history, dental history, and dental examination), before learning to critically evaluate the treatment options, to consider all factors that are relevant in the decision-making process, and to decide on the suitable options for discussion with the patient prior to reaching a clinical decision. Students were given sample patient case studies supplied by their disciplinary tutors (e.g. Figure 4.1), communicating the information orally in groups so as to boost students' competence in procedural vocabulary and to increase oral fluency.

AESTHETIC TREATMENT PLANNING PROBLEM

Case History:

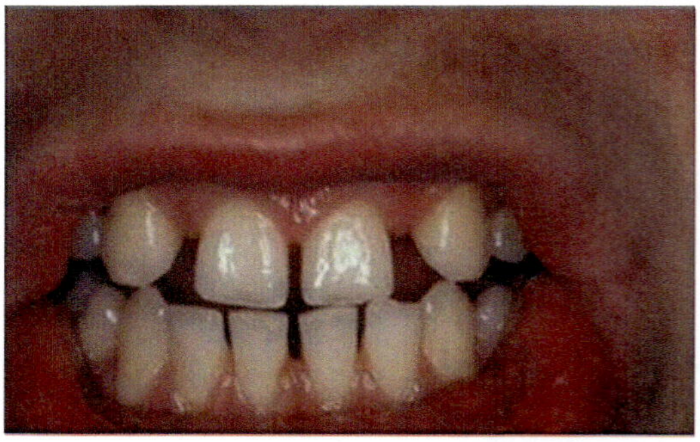

- A female patient aged 16 years presented with the congenital absence of 12 and 22.
- She was unhappy with the spaces between her upper anterior teeth.
- There was no relevant medical history.

Dental History:

- Father also has congenital absence of 12 and 22. No treatment had been received to correct the diastemas between his upper anterior teeth.
- Patient has just completed 18 months of orthodontic treatment to move the 13 and 23 distal to the 11 and 21 with a removable appliance. No movement to correct the midline diastema has been undertaken. The orthodontic retainer has not been worn.
- No restorations are necessary.

Dental Examination:

- The remaining permanent dentition was sound and the oral hygiene and periodontal status excellent.
- The upper midline labial frenum was attached to the palatal mucosa and a midline diastema of 1mm was noted.
- A diastema of 3mm was present between the upper right central incisor and canine, and of 4.5mm between the upper left central incisor and canine.
- The third permanent molar teeth were present on X-ray. Both 13 and 23 were slightly protrusive and the right canine was also angled distally.

Figure 4.1 Sample case study background for case report presentation

The change to the English-in-the-Discipline (ED) structure under the new four-year curriculum at HKU led to the end of direct instruction on case reports due to a new focus on the capstone *Community Health Projects* (Chapter 3). However, case reports are set to be re-implemented into the disciplinary curriculum in 2019 at the request of dental faculty supervisors. This will be in the form of *case-based learning*, an active learning strategy similar to problem-based learning which aims to expose students to a range of clinical situations in order to raise awareness of common clinical issues, dental problems and treatment strategies (Richards & Inglehart, 2006; Nadershahi, Bender, Lyon & Blaseio, 2013). Students will be trained in documenting the process and outcomes of clinical care before presenting them to other students and their disciplinary tutors. Empirical findings from a corpus of case reports would therefore offer valuable insights into final-year dentistry students' new needs in understanding the language of the clinical case report genre, as well as inform ESAP professionals when designing new course content.

A key methodological consideration for corpus linguistics is that it is sometimes preferable to approach a specialised corpus "to discover what is said about it, but to do so with as few constraining preconceptions as possible" (Murakami, Thompson, Hunston & Vajn, 2017: p. 244) as certain characteristics that could possibly be used to identify what is distinctive about our data can often lie hidden. As discussed in Chapter 1, there have been a number of corpus-based register analyses of medical case reports, with a smaller number of analyses specific to case reports in dentistry. These have looked at features including hedging and boosting devices (Salager-Meyer, 1991, 1994), narrative features and reference to person (Dorgeloh, 2016), structural features indicative of agency and identity (Schryer, Lingard, Spafford & Garwood, 2003) and pragmatic features (Kostenko, 2017). Rather than re-treading old ground by conducting similar analyses, the focus of this chapter is to consider the language of the case report genre from a different perspective without necessarily pre-determining what is selected for annotation (and what is not). The next section describes how this aim can be achieved through the use of natural language processing techniques (NLP), commenting on previous work in this area before we turn to our own analyses.

4.2 Natural language processing and ESAP

NLP refers to "the representation and automatic analysis and generation of human language" (Meurers, 2015: p. 537, c.f. Jurafsky & Martin, 2009). These can take the form of lexical, syntactic, semantic and pragmatic analyses according to the nature of the NLP procedures employed. Syntactic parsers and POS taggers make up the vast majority of applications used for corpus analyses, and are vital for the multidimensional analyses conducted in Chapters 2 and 3 of this volume. The use of automated semantic and pragmatic annotation of corpora is also commonplace within computational linguistics, and we are now beginning to see the use of these and other NLP tools in a range of applications related to language acquisition, including native language identification (e.g. Jarvis & Paquot, 2012), the estimation of L2 proficiency level (e.g. Pendar & Chappelle, 2008), the derivation of criterial features of proficiency levels (e.g. Hawkins & Buttery, 2010, Murakami, 2013), the dependency parsing of learner English (Lu, 2010; Huang, Murakami, Alexopoulou & Korhonen, 2018), and determining the variation in linguistic features that result from the effects of task complexity (Alexopoulou, Michel, Murakami, & Meurers, 2017).

NLP studies involving the derivation of target language features to be learned include the automated discovery of appropriate course reading materials (Ott & Meurers, 2010) and the automatic generation of language learning exercises (Aldabe, 2011). For academic English, NLP studies have explored the use of topic modelling (the automatic identification of sequences of text representative of the 'aboutness' of that sequence), with a view to training student writers to acquire these sequences (Murakami, Thompson, Hunston & Vajn, 2017). Other studies have employed machine learning to create an online collocation assistant for academic writing (Wu, Chang, Mitamura, & Chang, 2010); the construction of an intelligent automatic question generator for the purposes of automated written corrective feedback on academic writing (Lui, Calvo & Rus, 2012); the use of incremental parsers to aggregate analytics of the key features of academic writing for the purposes of displaying these analytics in a visual format for students (Simsek, Shum, De Liddo, Ferguson, & Sándor, 2014); and a wide range of studies on automated plagiarism detection (e.g. Barrón-Cedeño, Vila, Martí, & Rosso, 2013).

However, the number of NLP-based studies on disciplinary writing is much lower. One excellent exception is found in Crossley, Russell, Kyle and Römer (2017), who employed NLP tools that can measure lexical sophistication (TAALES, Kyle & Crossley, 2015) and cohesion indices (TAACO, Crossley, Kyle & McNamara, 2016) on the Michigan Corpus of Upper-Level Student Papers (MICUSP, Römer & Swales, 2010), a corpus composed of learner data from a range of disciplinary fields. These indices were compared across science and engineering papers as well as sub-fields within science and engineering, revealing significant cross- and within-disciplinary variation. Another exception is found in Yu and Zhang (2015), who used NLP tools to automatically derive disciplinary variation in authors' evaluative expressions within the context of academic citation practices. Comparing this function across the natural sciences and engineering disciplines, significant disciplinary variation was found in the purpose (e.g. comparison, critique) and polarity (e.g. positive, negative) of the citations present. Another brilliant example is found in Yan, Williams and Chen (2017), who used a domain-independent vocabulary extraction method on a large multi-disciplinary corpus, noting a power-law pattern in the frequency distributions of disciplinary vocabulary, which can be used in the future to automatically determine which discipline a given text was written for. Yan et al. however note that a good deal of NLP research on disciplinary writing is done at the metadata rather than whole text level. It is therefore our purpose in this volume to expand the use of NLP for investigating disciplinary writing to that of the dentistry discipline.

4.3 Constructing a corpus of case reports

We must state here that our original goal for this chapter was to compare professional case reports with novice undergraduate writing of such reports. This data would have allowed us to determine to what extent the novice writers were using the structures and lexis of professional case reports, and what more needed to be learned through ESAP so as to improve learners' writing. Despite receiving ethical approval from the Faculty of Arts to collect undergraduate attempts at case reports, disciplinary tutors in dentistry were eventually unable to provide us with this data as the anonymisation process could not ensure that patients would not be re-identifiable from the stored data. We are therefore restricted in this chapter to the analysis of professionally-written case reports in the hope of gaining teachable insights from this disciplinary genre that can be passed on to our ESAP cohort.

The data for the professional case report corpus is taken from the online, open-access, English-language journal *Case Reports in Dentistry*, which while not a highly ranked journal in the field (it is however indexed in the Clarivate Emerging Sources Citation Index), this journal was selected as it contains texts exclusively from the dentistry case report genre. The journal, according to its website, "publishes case reports in all areas of dentistry, including periodontal diseases, dental implants, oral pathology, as well as oral and maxillofacial surgery" (n.d.). Each submission adheres to strict structural requirements, and must include an abstract (of no more than 200 words) and an introductory section. Following the introduction, the 'case presentation' section is used (as stated in the author guidelines) to "present all of the relevant information about the patient in the case being reported, as well as a full description of the patient's symptoms, diagnosis, treatment, and outcome" (n.d.). This is followed by a discussion section which "should provide context for the case being reported and provide any necessary explanation of specific treatment decisions" (n.d.). There does not appear to be a word count requirement for articles in this journal, except for the abstract.

A research assistant downloaded all case reports published on the website since the journal's inception in 2011 to near the end of 2017, converting the reports into plain text files from their native HTML format, before manually clearing all boilerplate text, figures, images, tables, references, footnotes, and other extraneous information from the texts to leave only the running text and headings. The final corpus included a total of 810 case report articles, spanning 1,381,172 words of running text.

4.4 "Fear and disgust": A sentiment analysis of dental case reports

Our first investigation in this chapter involves a sentiment analysis of our case report corpus against that of the corpus of dentistry research articles featured in Chapter 2, using the *Sentiment Analysis and Cognition Engine* (*SEANCE*, Crossley, Kyle & McNamara, 2017). [21] A sentiment analysis involves the use of NLP procedures in determining the attitude, polarity and emotional content of the target text. While typically used in computational linguistics to derive opinions from the web for the purposes of marketing, public relations, and brand positioning (Pang & Lee, 2008), sentiment analysis is also finding its way into applied linguistics research. Much recent work has been done using sentiment analysis with corpora of tweets (Pak & Paroubek, 2010; Agarwal, Xie, Vovsha, Rambow, & Passonneau, 2011), as well as investigations into how expressions of sentiment can be used by companies to manipulate online reviews of their products (Hu, Bose, Koh, & Liu, 2012), but there has been precious little work on sentiment analysis for the study of academic writing. What work has been done has focused solely on the sentiment of citation practices, with Small (2011) running sentiment analysis on a multidisciplinary corpus, finding disciplinary variation in the form of sentiments employed, and with Athar (2011) identifying positive and negative sentiment as expressed in science writing, although neither of these studies had the express goal of developing disciplinary writing. It is therefore possible that our attempt here is the first such attempt to conduct a sentiment analysis of disciplinary texts for ESAP purposes.

Why conduct a sentiment analysis of case reports? As mentioned, the case report is the written documentation of real clinical interactions between dentists and patients. As noted by Schryer et al. (2003), it can be difficult for novice medical professionals to switch 'voices' from the non-clinical language that may typically be used in oral dentist/patient interactions, to that of the clinical dentist/dentist interactions as seen in the written case report, and vice versa. We assume these difficulties are compounded for L2 users who may be unaware of the different disciplinary and non-disciplinary senses of the lexis they are acquiring for case report writing. Students are likely to have acquired the non-disciplinary usage of the lexis of case reports *before* that of the disciplinary usage, which may make both the reading and writing of case reports difficult, at least in the early stages. It would therefore be useful for novice professionals to understand the range of non-disciplinary emotions and attitudes attached to the language of case reports, so that they can better understand the disciplinary usage when composing case reports of their own. Vice

21. https://www.linguisticanalysistools.org/seance.html

versa, this knowledge will also help novice dentists learn to switch 'voice' during dentist/patient interactions as they better understand the often powerful sentiment and emotions that disciplinary vocabulary may carry with it.

4.4.1 Procedure

SEANCE employs a "knowledge-based" method of sentiment analysis (Crossley, Kyle & McNamara, 2017: p. 810), classifying sentiment within a text by first POS tagging the data, then compiling affect categories (e.g. *fear*, *anger*) based on the frequency of particular affect words such as 'happy', 'sad', 'afraid', and 'bored' and other words with a probable affinity to particular emotions. These target words are contained in multiple wordlists such as the General Inquirer (Stone, Dunphy, Smith & Ogilvie, 1968), the Lasswell dictionary lists (Lasswell & Namenwirth, 1969) and the Hu and Liu (2004) polarity word lists.[22] *SEANCE* then analyses the corpus texts for the presence of words on these lists. Due to the large number of potential indices arising from this analysis (almost 3,000), *SEANCE* conducts a principle component analysis (PCA) on the dataset to reduce the number of indices selected from *SEANCE* to a smaller set of just twenty individual components, with resulting scores standardized across these components to facilitate comparison. The 20 components include *positive/negative adjectives, positive nouns/verbs, social order, action, joy, affect, fear and disgust, politeness, polarity nouns/verbs, virtue adverbs, respect, trust, failure, well-being, economy,* and *certainty*. We ran the *SEANCE* analysis on both the case report corpus, and the corpus of dentistry experimental research articles outlined in Chapter 2. Using the derived component scores across the two corpora, we used a stepwise (Wald) binary logistic regression as the method of statistical analysis, with the case report corpus as the target corpus for the regression.

From the analysis, seven of the twenty component rhetorical features annotated by *SEANCE* were found as significant predictors of the case report corpus, with five positive predictors and two negative predictors (which were positive predictors of the research article corpus). The model had adequate predictive power (-2LL = 440.62, Nagelkerke R^2 = .376) and passed goodness-of-fit tests (Hosmer & Lemeshow χ^2 = 6.78, d.f. = 8, sig = .560). The contribution of each feature to the model is outlined in Table 4.1.

We will now discuss the positive predictors indicative of dentistry case report writing in turn. As *SEANCE* does not yet output data as to which individual words are involved with a sentiment component within a dataset, Kristopher Kyle

22. A complete list of the relevant wordlists for each affect category is provided in the *SEANCE* manual (http://www.kristopherkyle.com/seance.html)

Table 4.1 Sentiment categories in dentistry case reports and research articles.

Feature	Component Score Dentistry Research Articles	Component Score Dentistry Case Reports	β	Sig.	(exp)β effect size
Negative adjectives	−0.399	−0.050	1.14	<.001	3.15
Fear and disgust	0.146	0.196	15.15	<.001	380.62
Positive nouns	−0.391	−0.205	4.13	<.001	62.34
Well-being	0.109	0.161	5.87	0.007	354.75
Positive verbs	0.04	0.001	0.77	0.012	2.17
-------	-------	-------	-------	-------	-------
Social order	0.291	0.281	−3.42	0.042	0.039
Economy	0.093	0.078	−10.58	<.001	0.000

gratefully provided the relevant wordlists via personal correspondence. Due to the massive number of words present in these wordlists, we used the freely available corpus analysis software *Coquery* (version 0.10, Kunter, 2017)[23] and loaded both the dentistry research report and case report corpora into the software. *Coquery* allows a user to search a corpus for the frequencies of search terms as embedded in a text file, allowing us to search for the frequencies of the thousands of terms in the wordlists related to the different sentiment categories involved in less than a minute. We then used the *Log-likelihood Calculator* (Rayson, 2016) to compare the keyness of individual terms from the wordlists across the two corpora.

4.4.2 Negative adjectives

For *negative adjectives*, the terms listed in Table 4.2 appear at least 30 times in the case report corpus and were considered after log-likelihood (LL) analysis as significantly more frequent within that corpus. Terms which could also have been coded as verbs (e.g. 'complete', 'correct') were not included in this list, as we cannot see the coded files. These terms all have an LL value of over 15.13 ($p < .0001$) and are ordered in Table 4.2 by their Bayes Information Criterion score (BIC, Wilson, 2013).[24]

23. https://www.coquery.org/

24. Bayes Factor can be interpreted as degrees of evidence against the null hypothesis (i.e. prevalence of terms are not different across corpora) as follows:

0–2: not worth more than a bare mention
2–6: positive evidence against H0
6–10: strong evidence against H0
> 10: very strong evidence against H0

Table 4.2 Negative adjectives in dentistry case reports / research articles

Word	Freq. case reports	Freq. research articles	Log-likelihood	Bayes factor BIC
malignant	382	5	112.78	98.45
foreign	327	9	75.70	61.37
traumatic	260	9	56.44	42.11
abnormal	222	6	51.81	37.48
aggressive	246	11	43.12	28.79
painful	108	1	34.18	19.85
chronic	541	56	33.13	18.80
superficial	105	1	33.07	18.73
inferior	254	16	32.94	18.61
immature	161	7	28.79	14.46
sterile	113	3	26.58	12.24
dominant	126	7	18.50	4.16
retrograde	43	0	16.76	2.42

Dentistry case reports are significantly more likely to include negative adjectives than experimental dentistry research reports. These are found in the 'case presentation' section, which often involves detailed descriptions of symptoms and conditions related to growths or cancers of the mouth, including 'malignant' and 'abnormal' , as well as scalar descriptions of pain, including 'painful' and 'chronic'. Importantly, there are a number of lexical items that have different senses in (non) academic/disciplinary contexts, and this is seen here with results such as 'sterile', 'foreign', 'superficial' and 'dominant'. It is therefore advisable to make L2 students aware of the different usages of these terms, so that they can disambiguate the appropriate sense of a term when encountering and using it in different contexts.

4.4.3 Fear and disgust

For *fear and disgust*, the terms listed in Table 4.3 appear at least 100 times in the case report corpus and were considered after analysis as significantly more frequent within that corpus. We have removed any items that also featured under the previous analysis for *negative adjectives* (i.e. 'aggressive').

It is again interesting to note here how the sense of an expression in the clinical sense can also be considered as a source of fear in non-clinical contexts. Terms that could be considered as neutral in terms of sentiment in clinical contexts such as 'diagnosis', 'examination', 'surgery', 'biopsy' and 'prognosis' also carry with them negative sentiments when viewed from the perspective of the patient, and novice dentists could be made aware of these differences both when dealing with patients (when the negative sentiment would apply) and when writing up case reports (when

Table 4.3 Features indicative of fear and disgust in dentistry case reports / research articles

Word	Freq. case reports	Freq. research articles	Log-likelihood	Bayes factor BIC
diagnosis	2,258	64	515.82	501.48
examination	2,268	119	350.40	336.07
swelling	928	8	297.29	282.96
cyst	779	4	267.29	252.96
tumor	775	7	246.36	232.02
surgery	1,423	81	204.28	189.95
pain	1,200	86	134.13	119.80
resection	374	4	115.28	100.95
eruption	565	21	111.89	97.55
cystic	375	5	110.24	95.90
biopsy	378	8	97.18	82.84
giant	339	10	76.00	61.66
prognosis	358	12	75.19	60.86
carcinoma	273	6	69.24	54.90
injury	341	15	60.48	46.15
bleeding	350	18	55.01	40.67
infection	685	64	51.36	37.03
recession	197	7	40.05	25.72
jaws	279	19	33.17	18.83
radiation	151	5	31.92	17.59
prevent	417	39	31.21	16.87
wound	217	14	27.42	13.09
damage	246	21	21.49	7.16

the disciplinary sense of these terms would apply). There are also significant genre differences in the frequency of these terms between case reports and research articles, presumably as case reports deal specifically with patients' clinical case presentation while research articles focus more on procedures (Chapter 2). As seen above, a number of terms within the case report corpus deal with growths, including 'swelling', 'cyst', 'tumor', 'eruption', 'cystic', 'giant', 'carcinoma', as well as injuries to the mouth including 'wound', 'bleeding', 'damage' and 'injury'. This appears to be indicative of the most frequent types of cases that dentists are involved with in their dental surgeries.

4.4.4 Well-being

For *well-being*, the terms listed in Table 4.4 appear at least 100 times in the case report corpus and were considered after analysis as specific to that corpus. We have removed any items that also featured under any previous analysis. Some of these are positive features of well-being, with some negative in polarity.

Table 4.4 Features indicative of +/− well-being in dentistry case reports / research articles

Word	Freq. case reports	Freq. research articles	Log-likelihood	Bayes factor BIC
patient	6,508	284	1,160.95	1,146.61
bone	4,062	393	285.36	271.02
trauma	787	30	153.48	139.14
gland	304	1	108.52	94.18
therapy	1,115	91	104.40	90.07
condition	677	63	63.28	48.95
vitality	175	3	48.15	33.81
discomfort	217	8	43.18	28.85
saline	180	9	28.95	14.62
sleep	104	2	27.61	13.28
surgeon	137	5	27.42	13.09
body	493	55	25.42	11.09

While *SEANCE* has categorised these expressions according to a general sense of well-being outside of a strictly clinical context, there are a number of terms that feature heavily in case report writing and which barely feature at all in research reports, the most significant of which is 'patient'. Unlike experimental research articles, which were shown in Chapter 2 to focus more strongly on procedures, there is a very strong focus on the patient in case report writing, a focus that can and should be communicated to novice writers of this genre. Various other terms are related to descriptions of the patient's attributes or conditions (e.g. 'condition', 'discomfort', 'vitality', 'body', 'sleep'). Reference to the dental surgeon themselves is also more likely to occur in case reports than seen in research articles.

4.4.5 Positive nouns and verbs

For *positive nouns* and *positive verbs*, the terms listed in Table 4.5 appear at least 30 times in the case reports corpus and were considered after analysis as significantly more frequent within that corpus. We have removed any items that also featured under any previous analysis.

Concordances of the term 'smile' were checked using *AntConc* to determine if they were being used as a noun. A cursory investigation of concordances determined that 'aspiration' was rarely used in a positive non-disciplinary sense (i.e. as a synonym for 'dream') in the corpus, although it is useful to make students aware of the different usages of such terms in different contexts. The patient-focused terms 'recovery' and 'improvement' are significantly more likely to appear in case report writing than in research reports. Case reports also frequently clarify that the procedures undertaken were a 'success', and also frequently list the advantages of particular treatment methodologies, with reports often detailing how dentists describe these advantages directly to patients prior to surgery.

Table 4.5 Positive nouns and verbs in dentistry case reports / research articles

Word	Freq. case reports	Freq. research articles	Log-likelihood	Bayes factor BIC
[Nouns]				
success	475	48	30.60	16.26
smile	164	7	29.71	15.38
aspiration	104	2	27.61	13.28
advantages	222	15	26.63	12.30
traction	85	1	25.69	11.36
recovery	78	1	23.13	8.80
improvement	226	18	21.93	7.59
[Verbs]				
like	601	40	73.37	59.03
advocated	60	1	16.64	2.31

4.5 Arts, crafts and dentistry? The semantic domains of dentistry case reports

Our next analysis of the case report corpus involves the use of a semantic tagger. Here, we employ the *UCREL Semantic Analysis System* (USAS, Rayson, Archer, Piao, & McEnery, 2004), available as part of the *Wmatrix* web-based corpus processing environment (Rayson, 2009).[25]

Why conduct a semantic analysis of case reports? As seen in the sentiment analysis reported in the previous section, it is evident that much of the vocabulary within case reports may have multiple senses according to disciplinary vs. non-disciplinary usage, and which contain an array of positive and negative attitudinal and emotional content that L2 learners in particular need to be able to recognise when reading and writing case reports. While the sentiment analysis generally deals with the polarity of this vocabulary, a semantic analysis can allow one to derive the different semantic domains from which these multiple senses are drawn. This is important because L2 students in particular may struggle to (dis) associate polysemous lexical meanings acquired in one domain to that of the target discipline, and vice versa, due to limited lexical knowledge of polysemy and a lack of disciplinary register/genre awareness of polysemous lexis in the target language. Students may not be aware of which lexical items within disciplinary texts have multiple senses across various semantic domains, nor be aware of how many semantic domains (other than 'science', for example) frequently criss-cross into disciplinary writing. This may make the initial reading and writing of case reports difficult for

25. http://ucrel.lancs.ac.uk/wmatrix/

novice L2-speaking disciplinary writers. By first discovering the different semantic domains that criss-cross into disciplinary writing, and then making disciplinary writing students aware of these multiple meanings through focused, corpus-based tasks, this (for us) is a novel variation on the derivation and use of academic word lists in the disciplinary writing classroom. Whiteside and Wharton (2019: p. 1) also suggest that from a practitioner's perspective, a corpus-based semantic approach "uncovers meaning-focused lexico-grammatical features of very high value due to their extremely regular occurrence within student texts", and that because of this high density of such semantic features, "a lexical approach to disciplinary language may be of particular value in the classroom" (p. 19).

4.5.1 Procedure

We uploaded the entire case report corpus to *Wmatrix*, where it was POS-tagged with the CLAWS tagger (Rayson & Garside, 1998), before USAS automatically tags each lexical item in the corpus across 21 possible discourse fields (see Figure 4.2).

A general and abstract terms	B the body and the individual	C arts and crafts	E emotion
F food and farming	G government and public	H architecture, housing and the home	I money and commerce in industry
K entertainment, sports and games	L life and living things	M movement, location, travel and transport	N numbers and measurement
O substances, materials, objects and equipment	P education	Q language and communication	S social actions, states and processes
T Times	W world and environment	X psychological actions, states and processes	Y science and technology
Z names and grammar			

Figure 4.2 USAS semantic domains annotated in *Wmatrix* (http://ucrel.lancs.ac.uk/usas/, n.d.)

These 21 fields are divided into hundreds of subcategories, a full list of which can be found by visiting the USAS homepage.[26] USAS then derives frequency lists of the tagged semantic domains present in the corpus, which can then be contrasted with another reference corpus built into Wmatrix. This approach builds on the typical cross-corpus keyword analysis technique employed in many contrastive lexical analyses, by applying keyness calculations to frequency lists of semantic tags. (Rayson, 2008). Rayson suggests that such an approach allows for the "macroscopic" analysis of whole texts (or in our case, texts representative of the case report genre) which can then inform a "microscopic" analysis of a particular semantic domain or linguistic features present within that genre, in this case combining the "corpus-based" and "corpus-driven" paradigms of corpus linguistics (Rayson, 2008: p. 519). This is another method whereby we can approach a specialised corpus without making *a priori* decisions about what to investigate (Murakami, Thompson, Hunston & Vajn, 2017).

Excluding the grammatical categories from the *Z:Names and grammar* domain (as shown in Figure 4.2) which include pronouns, particles, 'if', and other unmatched forms, words containing semantic information from these 21 fields were annotated 486,244 times within the corpus. Figure 4.3 shows the frequencies of these annotations across the semantic domains present within the case report corpus.

The results suggest that *general/abstract terms,* as well as terms related to *the body and the individual, numbers and measurement, substances/materials/objects and equipment, movement and location, psychological actions/states/processes, time,* and *social actions/states/processes* are highly frequent within the corpus with over 10,000 annotations each, accounting for 92.26% of the annotated semantic categories. Some of these domains can perhaps be considered closely related to dentistry (e.g. *the body and the individual* with reference to the anatomy of the mouth, or *substances/materials/objects* with reference to dental materials such as enamel, dentin). Interestingly, a number of the derived semantic domains that frequently occur in the case report corpus have less obvious semantic relations with dentistry *per se,* such as *movement and location, psychological actions/states/processes, time,* and *social actions/states/processes*. However, it is apparent from the results that a good deal of the vocabulary present within case report writing is derived from these semantic domains. This finding is important for ESAP provision, as no explicit instruction for making students aware of the importance of these domains within dentistry writing was previously found within the ESAP (or even EGAP) course materials. It is also interesting that there are not an inconsiderable number of annotations (in the low thousands) from semantic domains with no discernible link to dentistry such as

26. http://ucrel.lancs.ac.uk/usas/

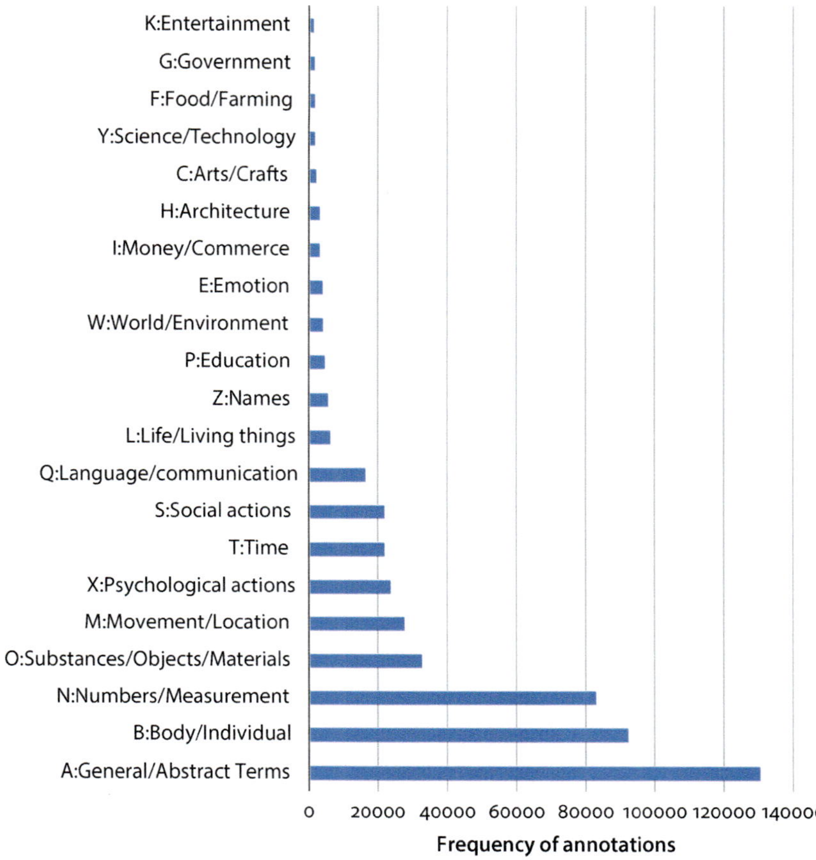

Figure 4.3 Frequency of semantic discourse fields within dentistry case reports

food and farming, *arts and crafts* and *money and commerce* within the case report corpus. Of course, it should be perfectly obvious that dentistry case reports do not discuss food and farming, although there do appear to be terms present within the case report corpus that could also have a sense that belongs to that domain, and it would be useful for L2 students in particular to be aware of these multiple usages if they are not already. However, the remainder of this chapter will focus only on the eight most frequently annotated domains.

Our next sets of analyses are therefore data-driven, using these corpus-based results as a starting point. We first present the keywords specific to the case report corpus according to each of the eight most frequently annotated semantic domains, before presenting the key subdomains specific to the dentistry corpus. To determine specificity in both cases, we compared the results above from our case report corpus with those derived from the *BNC Sampler Written*, which is a 1,000,000 word subset of the *British National Corpus*. Our choice to use the BNC Sampler over the corpus of experimental research articles (as used for the sentiment analysis) is a technical issue, as we were unable to upload this corpus into *Wmatrix* due to file size and format limitations. However, the *BNC Sampler Written* is freely available within *Wmatrix* as a reference corpus, and as this corpus is representative of a general range of written registers, this makes a useful point of comparison for a specialised disciplinary corpus (such as our corpus of case reports). *Wmatrix* then performs log-likelihood calculations on the frequency list of the annotated lexical items and semantic domains across both corpora in order to derive each corpus' key lexical items and key domains.

4.5.2 General and abstract terms

Beginning with *general and abstract terms,* Figure 4.4 describes the subdomains considered as more likely to be found within the case report genre as compared with their prevalence within the *BNC Sampler Written*. Each row represents a subdomain within *general and abstract terms* preceded by its accompanying USAS code. Certain subdomains can themselves have other subdomains, indicated by +/– values typically representative of their polarity. The value listed on the x-axis is that of the BIC effect size criterion score, representative of the keyness of a subdomain within the case report corpus as opposed to its presence in the *BNC Sampler Written*.

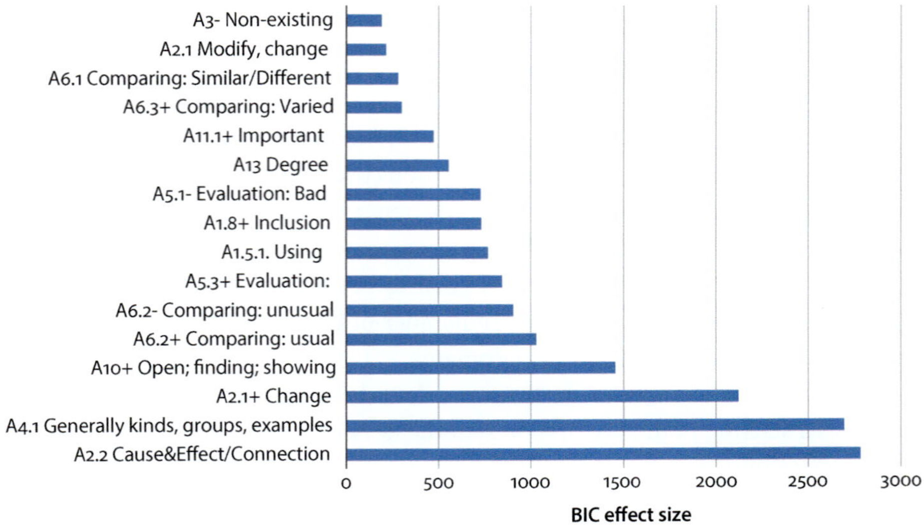

Figure 4.4 Key subdomains of **general and abstract terms** in the case report corpus

While all of these results exhibit very high BIC effect sizes for keyness, the subdomain most closely associated with the case report corpus is that of A2 *affect*, with A2.2 *cause & effect / connection* as the semantic subdomain most specific to case reports. Within this domain, the expressions 'due to' (n = 1026), 'result(s)' (n = 953), 'cause(d/s)' (n = 930), 'factors' (n = 420), 'because of' (n = 390), 'based on' (n = 358), 'related' (n = 276), 'resulting' (n = 233), 'lead to' (n = 196) and 'hence' (n = 195) are the ten most frequent examples of this subdomain within the case report corpus, representing the way that professional writers of case reports structure causation. This is mainly done in the description of the case symptoms, as well as when making recommendations for other dentists, either based on the procedure the authors had performed or with reference to established findings from the literature:

> Extraorally, there was a facial asymmetry due to bulging of the left cheek …
>
> The mass had caused displacement of zygomaticus major muscle and facial artery …
>
> An early and timely intervention would lead to better management of transmigrated canines.
>
> Direct cutdown on the stones in the longitudinal portion of the duct is ill advised as it can lead to the maceration of the duct making sialodochoplasty impossible and may result in salivary leakage or stenosis [9, 15, 16]

In addition, A2.1 (*modify, change*) and its subdomain A2.1+ (*change*) are also highly specific to the case report corpus, with the words 'restoration' (n=539), 'development' (n=436), 'restorations' (n=448), 'affected' (n=440), 'formation' (n=434), 'occur' (n=403), 'changes' (n=314), 'occurs' (n=267), 'occurrence' (n=253), and 'developmental' (n=185) as keywords specific to the case report corpus within that subdomain. 'Change' is a key element of the case report genre, found in the resolution, via surgery, of patients' dental complaints. 'Restoration(s)' of teeth feature heavily in the data, while 'occurs' features in descriptions of symptoms that are affected conditionally, and 'affected' is used to report on changes to the body or categories of patients as the result of disease or accident:

> Therefore, restoration of teeth after endodontic treatment is becoming an integral part of the restorative practice in dentistry …
>
> This re-eruption occurs especially when the dental pulp is vital, and hardly occurs when pulp necrosis is established [14]
>
> Other areas to be commonly affected are palms, soles, lips, oral mucus membrane, and conjunctiva …

Another key domain specific to the case report corpus was that of A6 *comparing*, with the subdomains A6.2+ *comparing: usual*, A6.2- *comparing: unusual*, A6.1 *comparing: similar/different* and A6.3+ *comparing: varied* all within the 15 semantic sub-domains most specific to the case report corpus. Within *comparing: usual*, the words 'normal' (n = 855), 'common' (n = 592), 'usually' (n = 571), 'commonly' (n = 351), 'conventional' (n = 322), 'natural' (n = 176), 'generally' (n = 168), 'routine' (n = 157) and 'regular' (n = 125) all appeared over 100 times within the case report corpus, while for the subdomain *comparing: unusual*, the words 'unusual' (n = 204), 'dysplasia' (n = 199), 'abnormalities' (n = 167), 'anomalies' (n = 164), 'abnormal' (n = 159), 'anomaly' (n = 146) and 'uncommon' (n = 111) all appeared over 100 times in the data. 'Normal' was particularly productive, found to collocate frequently with limits, ranges, appearances and development:

> Patient's complete hemogram was done and all the parameters were found to be within normal limits.
>
> Mandibular movements were in the normal range …
>
> Skin and nails were of normal appearance …
>
> Intraoral examination showed normal development of the dentition …

For *comparing: similar/different*, the lemma 'compare(d)' (n = 267) occurred frequently, while for *comparing: varied*, the words 'various' (n = 330), 'variations' (n = 168), 'combination' (n = 150) and 'mixed' (n = 105) all appeared over 100 times in the case report corpus data. 'Compared' most frequently collocated with 'to', and was used when comparing findings from the literature, or when comparing the characteristics of dental features or symptoms. 'Various' was used to describe treatments, other studies and methods:

> Children in particular are more likely to experience dog-bite injuries compared to adults …
>
> There was fullness of face on the right side as compared to the left side …
>
> Various treatment methods have been proposed to correct anterior dental crossbite …
>
> It has been shown by various studies on HIV and AIDS that oral candidiasis is the most common opportunistic infection [2, 4]
>
> Various methods and techniques were employed to restore fractured teeth which include pin retained resin, orthodontic bands, stainless steel crowns, porcelain jacket crowns, and complex ceramic restorations [11, 12].

The domain A4.1 *generally kinds, groups, examples* featured heavily in the case report corpus. Within this domain, the words 'case(s)' (n = 4769), 'type(s)' (n = 822), 'side' (n = 322), 'characterised' (n = 265), 'form' (n = 225), 'aspect' (n = 186), 'definitive' (n = 162), 'classified' (n = 139), 'classification' (n = 131) and 'specimen' (n = 120) were the ten most frequent items. 'Case' obviously collocated with 'case report', but also with 'of', typically in the abstract. 'Types' also frequently collocated with 'of', and is used to describe complex conditions, while 'characterised by' was another frequent construction in the corpus, used when explaining the common symptoms of a condition.

> We report a case of peripheral ossifying fibroma overlying the mandibular alveolar ridge of a 55-year-old female ...
>
> This report describes the case of an 8-year-old boy that was referred to endodontic and orthodontic treatment ...
>
> According to Jones, there are three types of hypodontia which include mild (1 or 2 teeth missing), moderate (3–5 teeth missing), and severe (above 6 teeth missing) [13].
>
> Hutchinson-Gilford progeria syndrome (HGPS) is a rare paediatric genetic syndrome with incidence of one per eight million live births. The disorder is characterised by premature aging, generally leading to death at approximately 13.4 years of age ...

A5.3+ *evaluation* and A5.1- *evaluation: bad* were also key semantic subdomains within the case report corpus, with the words 'right' (n = 757), 'correct' (n = 209), 'correction' (n = 159) and 'accurate' (n = 121) appearing within *evaluation*, and the words 'defect(s)' (n = 561), 'severe' (n = 486), and 'severely' (n = 103) under *evaluation: bad* also appearing more than 100 times within the data. However, 'right' is rarely used for evaluation in the corpus, primarily being used in its locative sense. 'Correct' is typically used as a verb, but it is often used to evaluate diagnoses and treatments. A 'defect' in dentistry is a term to describe an abnormality of a dental feature, while 'severe' was most frequently used to describe pain or symptoms.

> Knowledge about the anatomy of the root canal system is essential for successful endodontic therapy and permits a correct diagnosis followed by thorough cleaning and shaping of root canals [1, 2]
>
> A thorough physical, psychic, and social assessment is in order to provide the correct treatment [5].
>
> The resulting tissue defect was primarily closed with local flaps ...
>
> The patient was in severe pain as a result of a large pulp exposure.
>
> The prognosis of cracked tooth that is not treated will progressively deteriorate and may evolve into a split tooth or result in severe periodontal defects [1]

4.5.3 The body and the individual

Table 4.6 describes the subdomains associated with the case report corpus for the domain *the body and the individual.* For B1 *anatomy and physiology,* the ten most frequently occurring expressions within that domain were 'teeth' (n = 3612), 'tooth' (n = 2987), 'bone' (n = 2250), 'dental' (n = 2208), 'oral' (n = 1617), 'tissue' (n = 1363), 'cells' (n = 889), 'periodontal' (n = 818), 'incisors' (n = 737) and 'mouth' (n = 642), with all of these typically also used within dental research articles as well. Taking B2 *health and disease* and its subdomains together, the ten most frequently occurring expressions were 'patient(s)' (n = 5877), 'lesion(s)' (n = 2308), 'pain' (n = 747), 'syndrome' (n = 700), 'fracture' (n = 600), 'tumor' (n = 584), 'disease' (n = 569), 'cyst' (n = 474), 'infection' (n = 431) and 'symptoms' (n = 412), with all of these for subdomain B2- *disease.* For B3 *medicines and medical treatment,* the ten most frequently occurring expressions were 'treatment' (n = 3725), 'clinical' (n = 2037), 'diagnosis' (n = 1478), 'surgical' (n = 1199), 'implant' (n = 1004), 'anterior' (n = 953), 'surgery' (n = 789), 'therapy' (n = 646), 'orthodontic' (n = 577) and 'extraction' (n = 453) within this subdomain. Finally, for B4 *cleaning and personal care,* the words expressions 'tissues' (n = 561) and 'oral hygiene' (n = 340) appeared more than 100 times in the corpus, although 'tissues' was often a false positive involving paper tissues, rather than skin, muscle and nerves. Overall, these results are unsurprising as the extracted subdomains and lexical items are generally taken from medical terminology, although it is also interesting to see the domain of *cleaning and personal care* as a major semantic domain of dentistry case reports, presumably as a key component of the post-treatment advice given to patients following the clinical procedure.

Table 4.6 Key **body/individual** related subdomains within dentistry case reports

Domain field code	Domain subcategory label	Freq. case reports	Freq. BNC Sampler	Log-likelihood	Bayes factor BIC
B1	Anatomy and physiology	30,974	5,489	34,472.29	34,457.90
B3	Medicines and medical treatment	25,183	1,711	28,678.38	28,663.99
B2-	Disease	23,721	1,275	28,527.17	28,512.77
B2	Health and disease	626	129	445.03	430.63
B4	Cleaning and personal care	1,679	883	403.25	388.86
B2+	Healthy	310	195	49.3	34.9

4.5.4 Numbers and measurement

Table 4.7 describes the 10 subdomains of *numbers and measurement* most common found within the case report corpus data. There was much more frequent use of N1 *numbers* in the case report corpus than in the BNC. The main semantic focus of the case report data for this discourse field is that of N3 *measurement,* including measurement of *area, distance, length and height*, each of which feature heavily in the data during recounts of surgical procedures and analyses of patient conditions. For *measurement* generally, the word 'molar' occurs 216 times, although this is likely to be a false positive as this refers to the teeth rather than the unit of measurement. For measurement of *area*, the word 'space(s)' (n = 521) occurs frequently for this function, while for measurement of *distance*, the abbreviations 'mm' (n = 1,025) and 'cm' (n = 318) occur frequently, as do the words 'extending' (n = 170) and 'range' (n = 127). 'Space' commonly occurs as part of 'orthodontic space closure', which is a dental term for removing gaps in a patient's smile, and it is also commonly used in the description of a surgical procedure where one procedure makes space for another procedure to be conducted, while 'extending' is most frequently used to describe an extension from a specific area of the mouth, or to that area.

> Multibracket straightwire fixed appliance was used to open the space for dental implant placement, and treat the impaired occlusion.
>
> A pedunculated, rubbery, nontender, and pinkish mass of gingival-like tissue was seen extending from lower left first premolar to lower left second molar.
>
> Followup of the patient indicated bone necrosis on the anterior maxilla including the alveolar process extending to the palate …

Table 4.7 Key **numbers and measurement** related subdomains within dentistry case reports

Domain field code	Domain subcategory label	Freq. case reports	Freq. BNC Sampler	Log-likelihood	Bayes factor BIC
N1	Numbers	31,960	15,606	8,822.12	8,807.72
N5	Quantities	9,982	6,385	1,516.72	1,502.32
N5---	Quantities: Little	690	65	713.94	699.55
N6-	Infrequent	1,218	410	566.59	552.2
N3.6	Measurement: Area	566	93	461.26	446.87
N3.3	Measurement: Distance	2,077	1,411	264.43	250.04
N3	Measurement	231	20	245.63	231.23
N3.7	Measurement: Length and height	1,438	965	190.12	175.73
N3.6+	Spacious	153	27	119.8	105.4
N3.7-	Short and narrow	543	310	109.62	95.22

For measurement of *length and height*, the expressions 'length' (n = 237), 'level' (n = 202), 'diameter' (n = 195), 'thickness' (n = 179), 'height' (n = 156) 'width' (n = 120) and 'levels' (n = 114) all occur greater than 100 times in the data, and are typically used in descriptions of symptoms or surgical tools, or with 'level' typically used to describe the condition of bone or gingiva:

> Take two pieces of 0.014″ stainless steel (SS) wires of about 3.5 cm in length as "guide wires" …
>
> In Figure 4(d), the normal alveolar bone level after extraction is seen.

Quantities also feature heavily in the case report data, with the words 'both' (n = 623), 'figures' (n = 618), 'some' (n = 559), 'several' (n = 402), 'number' (n = 370), 'any' (n = 204), 'amount' (n = 158), 'portion' (n = 136), 'margin' (n = 129) and 'sufficient' (n = 125) the ten most frequent for *quantities* generally, and with 'less' (n = 175) appearing for *quantities: little*. 'Portion' appears to be used as a locative.

> The central portion of the hyoid bone …
>
> Anterior portion of right nasal cavity …

4.5.5 Substances, objects and materials

Figure 4.5 shows the subdomains of *Substances, objects and materials* deemed specific to the case report corpus. *Substances and materials* feature heavily in the case report data, both generally (O1) and in terms of *solid* and *liquid* substances/materials (O1.1/O1.2). For the *general* subdomain, the words 'material(s)' (n = 830), 'calcium' (n = 230), 'acrylic' (n = 181), 'acid' (n = 150), 'hydroxide' (n = 131), 'collagen' (n = 106) and 'calcification' (n = 103) all occur greater than 100 times in the data, while for *solid* substances the words 'enamel' (n = 460), 'resin' (n = 456), 'gingiva' (n = 324), 'fibrous' (n = 247), 'cement' (n = 187), 'ceramic' (n = 178), 'metal' (n = 165), 'titanium' (n = 130), 'sodium' (n = 129) and 'porcelain' (n = 100) all occur greater than 100 times in the data. For *liquids*, the words 'pulp' (n = 669), 'water' (n = 102) and 'saline' (n = 101) all occur more than 100 times. These are all commonly used substances in dental clinical procedures, again suggesting the USAS analysis has accurately determined the specificity of the case report genre as compared with the general *BNC Written Sampler*.

The other main semantic subdomain specific to the case report corpus here is that of *physical attributes* (O4), of which *general appearance and physical properties*, *texture* and *shape* feature heavily in the data. For *general appearance and physical properties*, the words 'condition(s)' (n = 634), 'features' (n = 457), 'structure(s)' (n = 447), 'composite' (n = 402), 'presentation' (n = 267), 'excision' (n = 214), 'bony'

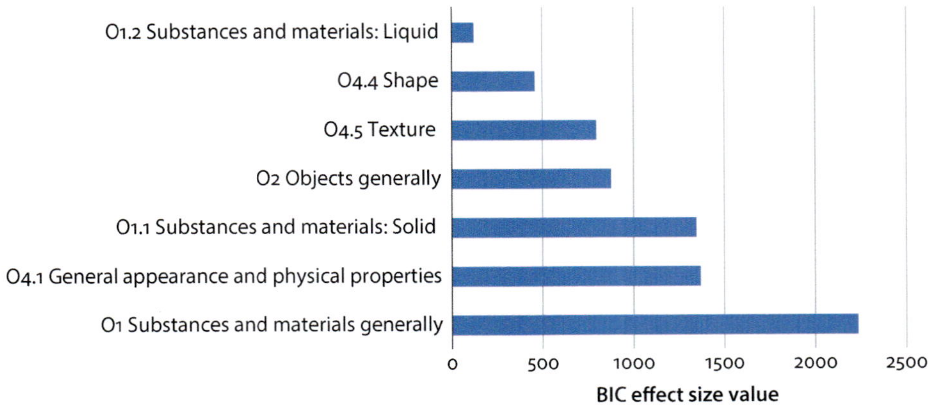

Figure 4.5 Key subdomains of **substances, objects and materials** in the case report corpus

(n = 192), 'images' (n = 181), 'characteristics' (n = 162) and 'adhesive' (n = 112) are the ten most frequently occurring within that domain. 'Condition' is used to describe the well-being of a patient as a whole, but is more often used to describe a dental feature, or to describe an illness.

> The general health condition of the patient before the surgery was good …
>
> The choice is dependent on the condition of the remaining teeth …
>
> The osteomyelitis is an inflammatory condition of the bone …

'Presentation' is another interesting case, appearing in dentistry to be used similarly to 'condition' (most often preceded by the adjective 'clinical'), rather than in the sense of 'giving a presentation'.

> The clinical presentation of the gingiva was similar to that of hereditary gingival hyperplasia but did not have a contributory medical or family history [1–3]
>
> This paper presents a report of 2 cases of Papillon-lefevre syndrome in which diagnosis is based on clinical presentation and genetic mapping …

For *shape* the words 'vertical' (n = 259), 'midline' (n = 199), 'shape' (n = 191), 'angle' (n = 160), 'horizontal' (n = 158), 'line' (n = 153) and '3d' (n = 129) all appear over 100 times in the data. 'Midline' is a medical locative term relating to a median line or plane of bilateral symmetry. This term is often found as part of the condition 'midline diastema', which is a space or gap between the maxillary central incisors. The words 'soft' (n = 721), 'palatal' (n = 395) and 'hard' (n = 264) also occurred frequently for the subdomain *texture*, although in dentistry is appears to be used as a noun modifier, expressing location.

> It was believed that the cross-section of the mandibular impression paste was not wide enough in the midline and that this would negatively affect the stability of the right and the left tray pieces …
>
> Soft tissue examination revealed a wide midline diastema and hypoplastic labial frenum …
>
> The fracture line was oblique extending in apical direction from labial to palatal surface …

4.5.6 Movement, location, travel and transport

Only one specific subdomain within this superordinate domain was associated with the case report corpus – *location and direction* -with the others being specific to the BNC Sampler. The words 'this' (n = 2,844), 'lower' (n = 821), 'left' (n = 812), 'presence' (n = 774), 'mandible' (n = 767), 'upper' (n = 664), 'lateral' (n = 616), 'surface' (n = 614), 'posterior' (n = 559), and 'position' (n = 373) were the ten most frequent terms associated with this semantic domain within the case report corpus. Nouns frequently associated with 'lower' and 'upper' included 'lip', 'incisors', 'left', 'right', 'arch', 'anterior' and 'jaw', while 'incisor' was the main noun associated with 'lateral', and 'teeth', 'region', 'crossbite' and 'mandible' were frequent n-grams of 'posterior'. 'Presence' is invariably found within the construction '*the presence of X*', with 'teeth', 'canals', 'root' and 'cells' frequent collocates in the X position:

> Examination of teeth revealed presence of only nine erupted permanent teeth –17, 16, 13, 11, 21, 26, 27, 36, and 46 …
>
> Although Stroner et al. [3] have reported the presence of three distal canals in mandibular first molar as early as 1984 …

4.5.7 Psychological actions, states and processes

Table 4.8 describes the semantic subdomains more likely to be found within the case report corpus for *psychological actions, states and processes*. Subdomains with X3 *sensory* attributes feature twice in this list, namely *sound: loud* and *seen*. However, there appears to be a false positive for 'swelling' (n = 581) which has been annotated as a loud sound, leaving no other candidates for this subdomain. The word 'noticed' (n = 128) was the only word appearing frequently for the other sensory subdomain, *seen*. 'Noticed' was used frequently in reports of patient's descriptions of their symptoms, dentists' examinations and diagnoses, and descriptions of procedures:

> Five years later, the patient noticed mobility of the implant: the prosthesis was removed from the implant

Table 4.8 Key **psychological actions/states/processes** related subdomains within dentistry case reports

Domain field code	Domain subcategory label	Freq. case reports	Freq. BNC Sampler	Log-likelihood	Bayes factor BIC
X3.2+	Sound: Loud	587	52	619.68	605.29
X4.2	Mental object: Means, method	4,030	3,108	324.65	310.25
X9.2	Success and failure	271	51	204.2	189.81
X3.4+	Seen	160	53	75.76	61.36
X5.2++	Interested/excited/ energetic	71	13	54.4	40
X9.2-	Failure	459	369	30.76	16.36

> In addition, root fractures of the apical third of both maxillary central incisors were also noticed in the radiograph (Figure 1)
>
> Preauricular skin tags were noticed on both sides, with the left one being more prominent

An interesting finding is that a number of words occurred more than 100 times in the data for the subdomain *mental object: means, method*. Words within this subdomain relate to how an individual plans or maps what they are going to do, which appears to appear frequently in case report data. These words are 'procedure(s)' (n = 969), 'technique(s)' (n = 953), 'system(s)' (n = 408), 'approach' (n = 341), 'pattern' (n = 268), 'method(s)' (n = 232) and 'solution' (n = 119). Frequent modifiers of 'procedure' and 'technique' included 'surgical', 'impression' and 'apexification', while 'root canal', 'nervous', 'adhesive' and 'implant' were frequent modifiers of 'system'. 'Multidisciplinary', 'surgical', 'treatment', 'conservative' and 'intraoral' were the most frequent modifiers of 'approach', with 'growth', 'wax' and 'skeleton' frequent modifiers of 'pattern'. 'Methods' were frequently modified with 'conventional, 'treatment' and 'conservative', while 'saline', 'hypochlorite' and 'sodium' were frequent modifiers of 'solution', suggesting that the 'solution' is used to describe substances rather than methods in dentistry writing.

An additional interesting finding is that of a prevalence of terms related to *success and failure*, with the word 'outcome' (n = 186) frequently used to express success and failure generally, and with 'failure' (n = 212) used to express *failure*. This was also found in the sentiment analysis earlier in this chapter.

4.5.8 Time

Table 4.9 describes the semantic subdomains specific to the case report corpus for the field of *Time*. There is frequent reference within the case report corpus to *periods* of time, both generally as well as *long* and *short* periods of time. The word 'appointment' (n = 124) appears for the general subdomain, while 'deciduous' (n = 210), 'short' (n = 196) and 'provisional' (n = 166) feature more than 100 times for *short* periods of time, with 'chronic' (n = 382) and 'long term' (n = 167) feature more than 100 times for when describing *long* periods. The word 'permanent' (n = 703) is the only term frequently occurring for the *beginning* subdomain, with 'age' (n = 409) the only term for the *age* subdomain and 'early' (n = 476) for the *early* subdomain. Time expressions such as 'deciduous' and 'permanent' here mainly related to descriptions of child/adult teeth respectively, including 'canines', 'molars', 'dentition', etc.

Table 4.9 Key **time** related subdomains within dentistry case reports

Domain field code	Domain subcategory label	Freq. case reports	Freq. BNC Sampler	Log-likelihood	Bayes factor BIC
T2+++	Beginning	721	150	509.29	494.9
T3	Old, new and young: Age	1,368	722	326.25	311.85
T1.3-	Period: short	647	341	154.73	140.33
T1.1	General	181	47	108.18	93.79
T4+	Early	549	367	73.44	59.04
T1.3+	Period: long	801	733	25.25	10.86

4.5.9 Social actions, states and processes

Figure 4.6 shows the semantic subdomains of *social actions, states and processes* more frequently found within the dentistry case report corpus as compared with the *BNC Sampler Written*. S1.2 *personality traits* appear to feature frequently within the case report corpus, both generally and *informal/friendly* and *weak* traits specifically. The word 'immature' (n = 93) is the only trait to appear for the general subdomain with this use restricted to the phrase 'immature permanent teeth'. 'Fibroma' (n = 310) and 'benign' (n = 286) are listed as traits for the *informal/friendly* subdomain, and 'mild' (n = 193) as the only trait under *weak*, and these all have quite different senses in the dentistry discipline as compared with their usage to denote social states.

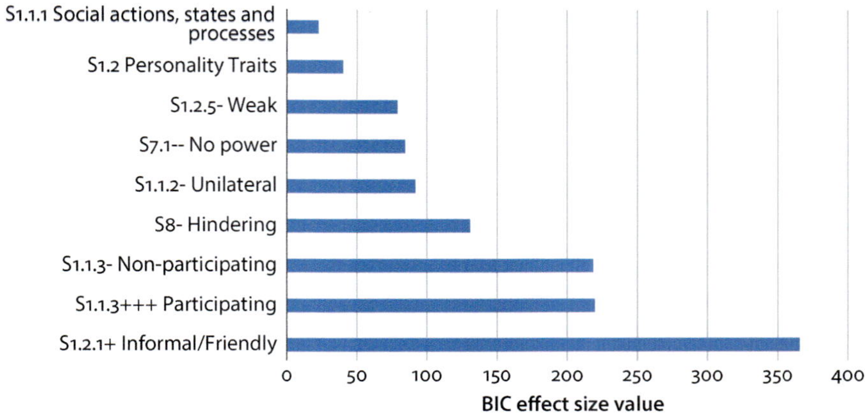

Figure 4.6 Key subdomains of **social actions/states/processes** in the case report corpus

Participating is also a key feature of the case report data, with variations of the word 'interfere' (n = 121) found for *participating* and 'absence' (n = 336) frequently found for *non-participating*. Again, these appear to have different senses in dentistry, with 'interfere' typically used when discussing 'development', and 'with 'absence' used when discussing missing teeth or symptoms, or when reporting on a positive outcome to a clinical procedure.

> This type of prosthesis allows the restoration of function and aesthetics of missing teeth and does not interfere with bone development …
>
> The successful result of this case was verified by the absence of clinical symptoms and by follow-up radiographs after 3 and 1/2 years (Figures 6, 7, and 8).

4.5.10 Combined semantic subdomains specific to dentistry case reports

Table 4.10 below describes the top 25 semantic subdomains across all semantic fields deemed significantly more likely to appear in dentistry case reports as compared with data of general written English from the *BNC Sampler Written*. The list was determined and organised according to Bayes factor BIC.

It is again interesting to note that aside from obvious dentistry relevant categories such as B3 *medicines and medical treatment,* B2 *health and disease* or B1 *anatomy and physiology* that each have over 20,000 annotations, there are a number of other semantic sub-domains that might not ordinarily be considered as specific to dentistry case reports but are statistically far more prevalent in these case reports than in general written English. Under the main field of *general and abstract terms* (A), the word 'missing' (n = 180) under the domain of A3- *non-existing* features

Table 4.10. Top key semantic subdomains specific to dentistry case reports

Domain field code	Domain subcategory label	Freq. case reports	Freq. BNC Sampler	Log-likelihood	Bayes factor BIC
B2-	Disease	23,721	1,275	28,527.17	2,100.85
B3	Medicines and medical treatment	25,183	1,711	28,678.38	1,641.10
A3-	Non-existing	187	14	207.53	1,480.08
N3	Measurement	231	20	245.63	1,266.31
X3.2+	Sound: Loud	587	52	619.68	1,235.37
N5---	Quantities: Little	690	65	713.94	1,155.75
A6.1	Comparing: Similar/ Different	300	32	297.08	1,009.02
A2.1	Modify/change	256	34	231.76	790.69
B1	Anatomy and Physiology	39,074	5,489	34,472.29	742.10
N3.6	Measurement: Area	566	93	461.26	619.95
N3.6+	Spacious	153	27	119.80	570.34
X5.2++	Interested/excited/ energetic	71	13	54.40	546.07
X9.2	Success and failure	271	51	204.20	528.59
S5+++	Belonging to a group	21	4	15.71	521.05
S1.1.2-	Unilateral	146	29	106.33	495.55
S7.1--	No power	138	28	99.12	483.03
B2	Health and disease	626	129	445.03	474.05
T2+++	Time: Beginning	721	150	509.29	468.61
O1	Substances and materials generally	3,235	689	2,248.79	455.42
T1.1	Time: General	181	47	108.18	355.56
S1.1.3-	Non-participating	417	117	232.93	321.62
A5.3+	Evaluation: Accurate	1,722	544	857.37	274.46
X3.4+	Seen	160	53	75.76	257.12
A11.1+++	Important	283	95	132.05	252.39
N6-	Infrequent	1,218	410	566.59	251.42

heavily in the data, as do the words 'compared' (n = 257) under the domain A6.1 *comparing: similar/different*; 'retraction' (n = 98) and 'calcified' (n = 52) under the domain A2.1 *modify/change*; 'right' (n = 757), 'correct' (n = 209), 'correction' (n = 159) and 'accurate' (n = 121) under the domain A5.3+ *evaluation: accurate*; and 'prevalence' (n = 211) under the domain A11.1+++ *important*. Likewise, under the main semantic field *numbers and measurement* (N), the words 'space' (n = 435), 'diffuse' (n = 106) and 'dilated' (n = 46) feature heavily under the subdomain N3.6

measurement: area; the words 'single' (n = 296), 'minimal' (n = 146), 'unique' (n = 66), 'minimise' (n = 66) and 'minimum' (n = 49) feature under the domain N5-- *quantities: little*; and the words 'incidence' (n = 230), 'sometimes' (n = 127) and 'frequency' (n = 96) occur frequently under the domain N6- *infrequent*.

The word 'permanent' (n = 703) is frequently found under the *time* subdomain *beginning*, with 'appointment(s)' (n = 124) under the *general time* subdomain. Under the domain *substances and materials generally*, the words 'material' (n = 589), 'materials' (n = 241), 'calcium' (n = 230), 'acrylic' (n = 181), 'acid' (n = 150), 'hydroxide' (n = 131), and 'collagen' (n = 106) all feature heavily in the case reports corpus. Words under the main semantic field *social actions and states* also feature heavily in the case report corpus. The word 'crowded' (n = 20) appears frequently under the subdomain *belonging to a group*; while the word 'unilateral' (n = 131) appears under *unilateral*; the word 'inferior' (n = 123) is frequent within the domain *no power*; and the word 'absence' (n = 336) appears frequently under the domain *non-participating*. Finally, under the main field of *psychological states and processes*, the word 'outcome' (n = 186) features frequently under the domain *success and failure*; while 'noticed' appears under the domain *seen*.

There were some false positives in the Wmatrix output however, with 'molar' appearing 216 times in the corpus under *measurement*; the word 'swelling' (n = 581) featuring under the subdomain of *sound: loud*; the word 'fixation' (n = 58) appearing under *interested/excited/energetic*, with these words having very different senses in dentistry than in their reported semantic domains for this analysis.

4.6 Scattertext and semantic domains

Returning now for a final comparison of the case report corpus and the experimental dentistry research article corpus from Chapter 2, we again ran the *Scattertext* (Kessler, 2017) software on the data to generate a graphic visualisation of keywords across both corpora (Figure 4.7). We mentioned in Chapter 2 that *Scattertext* uses a 'dense rank difference' method of determining corpus keyness in a visual output, with the x-axis 'indicating the rank of a word or bigram' along this axis in the reference corpus, with the same for the target corpus along the y-axis. The most frequent terms, regardless of ties, are ranked first on the axis, the next most frequent terms, regardless of ties, are ranked second, etc. Terms more associated with a particular corpus are a further distance from the diagonal line between the lower-left and upper-right corners, while terms are also coloured according to this distance.

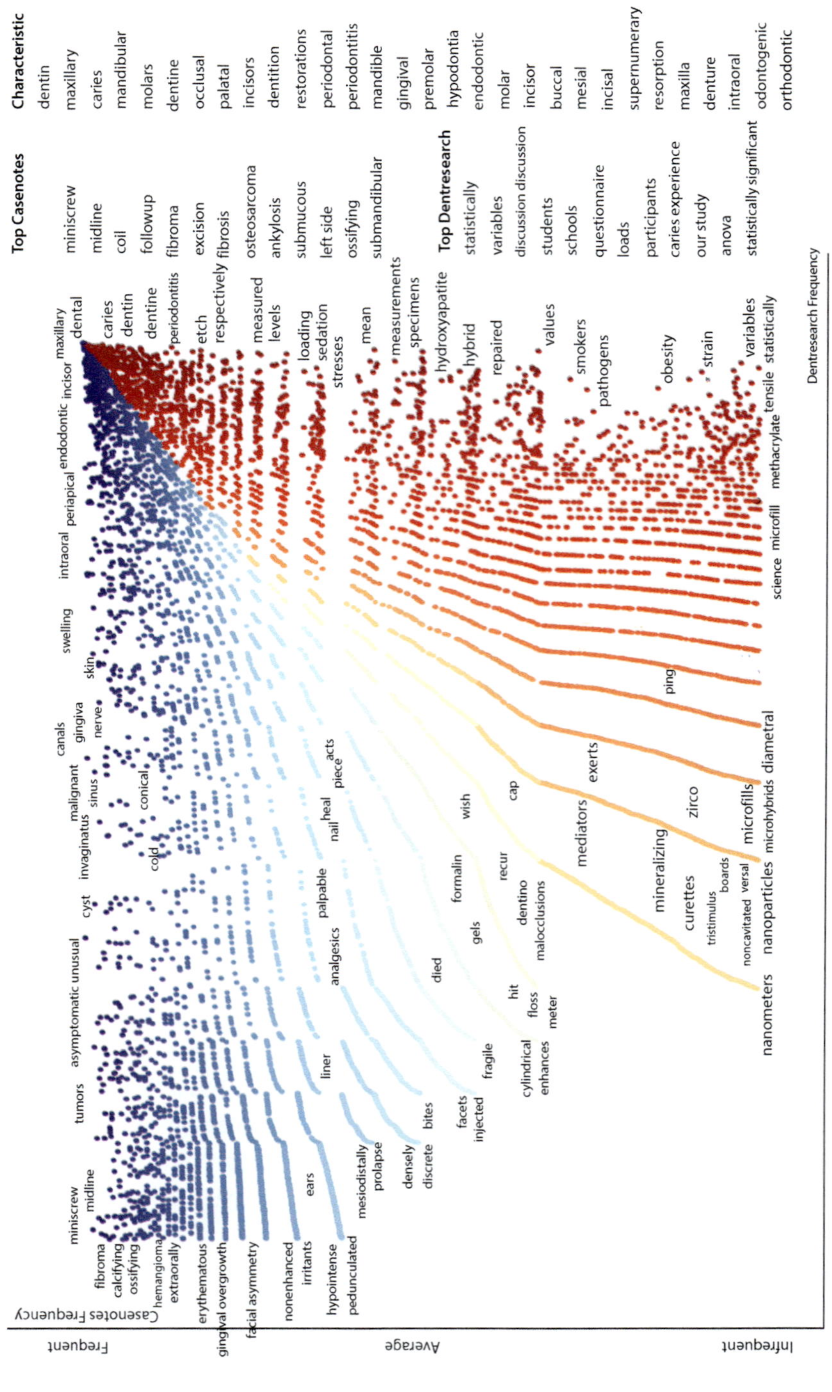

Figure 4.7 Scattertext of keywords across research report and case report genres of dentistry writing

Of interest, the top-ranked terms in the case report corpus come from a range of semantic domains. One such domain is that of adjectives describing the states/ conditions of patients or diseases, including 'erythematous' (redness of the skin caused by dilatation and congestion of the capillaries, often a sign of inflammation or infection), 'hypointense' (a 'less' intense abnormality on a magnetic resonance scan), and 'pedunculated' (where a mass such as a cyst or polyp is said to be pedunculated if it is supported by a peduncle, or an elongated stalk of tissue). Another domain is that of nouns referring to diseases and conditions, including 'osteosarcoma' (a common type of bone cancer), 'fibroma' (benign tumours) or 'hemangioma' (noncancerous growths of blood vessels). A third common domain is that of adjective modifiers of position to inform the reader as to the location of the symptom or where the procedure was carried out. These include 'mesiodistal' (a diameter joining the mesial and distal surfaces of a tooth), 'maxilliary left' (to the left of the pyramid-shaped maxillary sinus) and 'midline' (a median line or plane of bilateral symmetry). In contrast, the keywords of the dentistry research article corpus appear to be related to methodological and data reporting functions, including 'statistically significant', 'variables' and 'participants'. The words characteristic across both case report and research article corpora are very close to those seen in Chapter 2 for dentistry research articles vs. general medical research articles , including 'dentin', 'caries', 'mandibular', 'occlusal', etc. Therefore, while there are a lot of common vocabulary elements shared across both research report and case report genres of dentistry writing, the *Scattertext* analysis has shown that a number of semantic domains appear to be specific to the case report genre.

4.7 Chapter summary

In this chapter, we have revealed a number of insights into the lexical features of the dentistry case report genre via the use of automated NLP techniques, including sentiment and semantic analyses. The results and insights gained were both corpus-based and corpus-driven, as we approached the corpus analysis with as few preconceptions as possible, letting the numbers guide our exploration into the lexis used within dentistry case reports. We have found a wide range of terms that are typically used to convey positive and negative emotions in general English, and which are used in a more neutral, descriptive sense in dentistry writing. We have also seen significant differences in the use of these terms across the case report and research article genres in dentistry writing, which is highly suggestive of a particular focus on patients in the case report genre, as opposed to procedures in research articles. This is a surprising finding given that the function of case reports is that of reporting clinical procedures for dissemination among other dentists rather than for dissemination to the general public. We have also seen a wide range of lexical items within the case report genre that have alternative senses in other semantic domains, or are from semantic domains with a specific function in case report writing, such as measurement, comparisons, expressions of time, and descriptions of substances and methods. A number of lexical items within these domains were also compared across case report and research article genres using the Scattertext tool.

It is apparent from these findings that novice case report writers must be made aware of the different senses of the lexical items found here, and be able to recognise and switch between general and disciplinary senses of these items depending on their audience. For example, dentists may need to consider the general sense of an expression when in discussion with patients and the general public, and may also need to consider the sentiment of disciplinary lexical items during discussions – particularly if a term considered neutral in the dentistry discipline may be perceived as significantly negative in the general sense (e.g. 'malignant'). Vice versa, novice writers of any discipline should also be aware of the disciplinary rather than general senses of key terms when using them during disciplinary writing. This is particularly important for L2 learners who could be confused by these polysemous usages when both reading and writing disciplinary texts.

Additionally, our findings from the semantic domain analysis have revealed that there is a complex set of functions that each needs to be acquired to successfully complete specific stages of a complete case report. Writers must accurately describe states, materials, and patients' conditions using a vast array of disciplinary terminology, while precisely reporting on processes with specific reference to time, measurement, location, and movement. Similar findings regarding the discovery of latent semantic functions embedded in disciplinary writing using semantic tagging procedures have now been found in Whiteside and Wharton (2019) for texts spanning multiple disciplines, where "similarity far outweighed difference" (p. 18) in their cross-disciplinary usage (see also Durrant, 2017, for 4-grams and lexical bundles within history and politics disciplines). Given the high frequency of these semantic domains within the data, we argue that their associated functions appear to be hidden in plain sight, because they "have at their heart extremely, indeed unusually, frequent 'common' items" (Whiteside & Wharton, 2019: p. 18). It is highly likely that if we had only conducted a simple keyword analysis across dentistry and general written registers, or even dentistry case reports vs. research articles, we would have missed these vital functions of the case report genre in our analysis. Instead, via the adoption of a more corpus-driven approach, we have made these functions more salient when considering the requirements of the case report genre for novice writers. Of course, now that they are salient to us, it is our task to teach these functions to our novice writers. How we did this, and whether we succeeded in doing so, is now the focus of the second section of this volume.

SECTION II

Applying corpus insights for ESAP pedagogy

CHAPTER 5

Data-driven dentistry

Corpora, ESAP, and writing-to-learn

5.1 Introduction

This chapter explores the affordances of disciplinary corpora for ESAP materials development and data-driven learning pedagogy, with a specific focus on the integration of a purpose-built corpus query platform and accompanying corpus-based pedagogical activities into a 5th year undergraduate ESAP disciplinary writing course for dentistry. We first describe the rationale behind our adoption of a corpus-based approach for the teaching and learning of the complexities of grammar, disciplinary vocabulary, and rhetorical features as part of "writing-to-learn" for the discipline (Manchón, 2011) before explaining why our initial attempts to introduce disciplinary DDL pedagogy did not meet our expectations. We then describe the functionality of our online corpus query platform built to facilitate student exploration of the professional and learner corpora of Dental Public Health research reports outlined in Chapter 3. We explain how the findings from our analyses of research articles (Chapter 2), Public Dental Health articles (Chapter 3) and case reports (Chapter 4) drove the development of a suite of accompanying ESAP data-driven learning activities. The overall aim of this chapter is to show that with the right corpus platform and carefully structured accompanying activities, there is less need for students to have extensive technical skills and less need for teachers to devote time and effort on training students in corpus queries – both of which are claimed to result in teachers' reluctance to incorporate corpus-based data-driven learning into their practice (Leńko-Szymańska & Boulton, 2015).

5.2 The problem with 'learning-to-write'

Prior to the introduction of *English in the Discipline* (ED, see next section), the ESAP curriculum for dentistry followed a "learning-to-write" model (Manchón, 2011). There were two three-credit ESAP courses for dentistry students in the first year of the dental curriculum, one taken each semester. In the first semester, the curriculum focused on developing skills in oral English through in-class academic discussions and an oral presentation assessment based on a typical disciplinary problem supplied by the dentistry disciplinary tutors. For writing, the first semester curriculum aimed to train students to first cite and then critique published articles on selected topics in the dentistry domain. However, most activities in this first-semester course focused on the acquisition of medical and dental terminology, dealing with strategies in understanding word formation and word building skills so that students may quickly acquire a wealth of new medical and dental terminology. The second semester also contained both oral and written components, with the oral component involving simulated dentist-patient interactive role plays. The written component focused on the process writing of letters of referral and complaint and recognising the structural features of clinical case reports, achieved mainly via the use of exemplars with accompanying gap fill and matching activities. Most of the assessments and class time was taken up with the oral component of the curriculum, and the emphasis on writing primarily focused on activities dealing with local rather than global aspects of the referral letter and case report genres, despite the use of authentic exemplars. This approach, modelling the writing processes of the "good writer" while promoting the written text as an "object" for acquisition, sits firmly within the "learning-to-write" mode of writing instruction (Hyland, 2011).

While both courses received generally positive feedback from students and disciplinary tutors, the provision became increasingly disconnected from the revised dental curriculum resulting from the move from a 4 year to a 5 year curriculum and a new requirement to complete the Community Health Project (CHP) capstone in the fifth year of study. By the fifth year, senior dentistry students are required to demonstrate an advanced level of knowledge and competence in community dentistry through the completion of a supervised research project (the CHP), written in English. As the CHPs involve advanced study and research into the practice of preventive dentistry, oral epidemiology, and systems for the provision of dental health care and their administration, the ability to present the findings of this project require high communicative competence in English for academic reading, writing, and speaking. This meant the ESAP provision in year 1 now ran separately to rather than in tandem with students' disciplinary capstone projects, resulting in the ESAP content perceived as increasingly less important from both the dental students' and disciplinary tutors' perspectives. Despite building competence in the process writing of dentistry-specific genres, there were also no real opportunities for students to engage with the content of their writing, and no real opportunity for the writing activities to contribute to improved knowledge of the discipline. Having the ESAP provision in the first year also meant that a heavy focus on composition skills was considered unwelcome by freshman dental students, who were focusing on a busy schedule of experimental and clinical work from their disciplinary tutors during this period. Clearly, ESAP provision following the 'writing-to-learn' model wasn't going to cut it for much longer.

5.3 Corpora and 'writing-to-learn'

The shift to a new *English in the Discipline* (ED) format was that of a shift to 'writing-to-learn', with a new focus on getting students to become acquainted with disciplinary language features and discourse practices in order to "take on new roles and engage with knowledge in new ways" (Hyland, 2014: p. 142). Under this approach, students learn about the discipline through specially selected writing activities designed to reflect discipline-specific social practices and epistemologies. This process changes the nature of disciplinary and language content from that of "facts to be absorbed", as seen with the 'learning-to-write' model (Newell, 2008: p. 235). Rather, a more active, constructivist perspective is taken under the 'writing to learn' model, a switch to "knowledge-in-action" (Applebee, 1996: p. 16–17). To facilitate this switch, rather than being situated at the periphery, the ED course was for the first time offered in parallel to the capstone component of the five-year undergraduate program rather than in the freshman year, and aimed to offer concurrent language support during the final CHP, further enhancing fifth-year dentistry students' academic literacy for scientific research. During the course, students were to be guided in developing effective language skills in their written presentation of the CHP, and enhancing their ability to deliver a professional oral presentation of the project to their peers and disciplinary tutors (Schryer, Lingard, Spafford & Garwood, 2003). 3-hour sessions were conducted over 12 weeks of instruction covering the writing process, disciplinary language features and rhetorical devices of an entire scientific research report across the abstract, introduction, literature review, methods, results, discussion, recommendations, and conclusion sections, with ESAP provision in alignment with the respective stages of progress of the CHPs.

The use of corpora was crucial to the new ED provision from the outset. Given the new constructivist approach as featured under 'writing-to-learn', the role of the learner had now changed from a passive observer to "being in the driving seat" (Flowerdew, 2015: p. 18). This meant that the course materials needed to be able to promote the kind of higher-order cognitive processing and learner autonomy that students require to inductively make sense of multiple sources of data. Fortunately, the use of corpora under a data-driven learning approach is well-suited for promoting exactly this kind of learning (Chambers, 2007; Flowerdew, 2015), and the adoption of disciplinary corpora for this purpose would further enhance the learning to take place. Tribble (2001) suggests that novice writers need knowledge of content, the writing process, context, and the language system. According to Tribble, disciplinary corpora are particularly useful in aiding the acquisition of this knowledge, even more so when a professional reference corpus is combined with learner data, with both sources offering "essential information about the lexico-grammar, patterning and organisation which have made these texts allowable contributions to the genre" (2001, p. 381). From an ESAP tutor's point of view, while the development of course materials previously tended to rely on an intuitive sense of what students needed to learn (at least, without significant input from disciplinary tutors), the insights gained from corpora instead provided us with a range of authentic disciplinary language features both central to and cutting across key genres in dentistry. These insights allowed us to modify our existing course materials with new activities and exemplar texts containing a high degree of 'focus-on-form' (Long, 1991) for the acquisition of content knowledge, the writing process, and the language system. The disciplinary nature of the data also allowed us to meaningfully contextualise the language forms and meanings under investigation within the dentistry domain.

To facilitate this approach to learning more directly, we aimed to produce materials that would guide students into hands-on use of corpora as a key component of their overall disciplinary writing instruction. These activities would boost students' development of the technical, analytical and cognitive skills required to facilitate a "learner-centred" focus on form (e.g. Bernardini, 2001; Fuentes, 2017) under a true data-driven learning approach. Direct corpus use has been shown to be a catalyst for change in students' approaches to both L2 learning and L2 writing if training in this direct use is integrated within L2 writing courses, or at least running concurrently. As students gain more experience in writing, gain more experience using corpora, and gain more disciplinary/content knowledge, they are likely to express a qualitative sense of achievement in all three areas (Yoon, 2008). In fact, Yoon suggests "a focus on [disciplinary] content without taking into account their linguistic concerns may not lead them to become competent writers" (2008: p. 44).

5.4 Trial and error: First integration of corpora into ED provision

The 2016/17 course booklet introduces corpus-based learning as an "inquiry-based learning approach" (CAES9350 course materials, n.d.). In the introduction to the course's learning outcomes at the beginning of the booklet, students are informed that this means

> A unique feature of this course is to align with the faculty's inquiry-based and case-based approach by exposing you to 'real language problems' that academic writers face in research report writing. You will be exposed to specific language problems in real-life situations and will be instructed to consult professional and learner corpora to look for empirical evidence about language, enhancing your understanding of the complexities of disciplinary literacy (n.d.)

While the adoption of corpora to facilitate the switch to 'writing-to-learn' was now our goal, we had little time to prepare course materials involving corpora before the inauguration of dentistry ED in the 2016/2017 semester. Given this constraint, we were only able to create two activities requiring corpus consultation, with each involving the professional and learner corpora of Dental Public Health research reports that were the focus of Chapter 3. These activities were characterised as "language problem cases" in the materials, with one 'case' focusing on choosing the right tenses when reviewing the literature, and the other 'case' focusing on the use of hedging devices when making claims.

To facilitate these corpus tasks, we developed an online concordancer with access via the Moodle® learning management system that could allow students to query both the professional and learner Dental Public Health research reports outlined in Chapter 3. This was our first opportunity to work with a small team of computer scientists who had agreed to provide assistance as part of the university's *Technology-Enhanced Learning Initiative* (TELI), a centrally-funded initiative to provide technical support and innovation across a variety of projects. The user front-end and accompanying concordances for the query term 'dental' are shown in Figure 5.1.

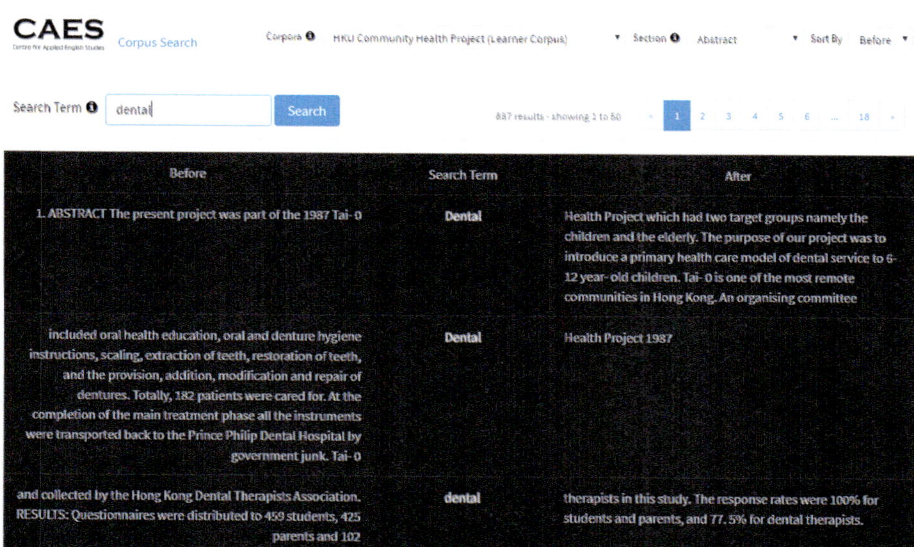

Figure 5.1 User interface for the 2016/17 corpus query platform

The platform allowed for users to produce simple corpus queries, without the option of filtering by POS, but including the possible use of wildcards. Only concordance output was displayed rather than any other visualisation of the data. Queries could be filtered by professional/learner corpora, and by section (e.g. abstract, literature review) in the learner corpus only. Users also had the option of sorting concordances before or after the query term, although only in alphabetical order rather than by a specific token.

In terms of learner training, a PowerPoint presentation was shown to students in class, containing some model activities where students could test the various functions of the corpus platform. This 2-hour session began with a comparison of dictionary output vs. concordance output. Students were invited to enter 'the data suggests that' into the website www.dictionary.com, and compare the null result there to concordance output generated by entering the same query term into the corpus platform. This activity was intended to 'sell' the corpus approach to students over their typical reference resources (see Chapter 6 for details of these). Next, students were asked to look for pre-modifiers of the query term 'research' by consulting the concordances to the left of the query term, and other words that 'research' could modify by consulting concordances to the right of the query term. Students were then invited to enter 'studies' as a query, sort concordances to the right, then locate any verbs in the concordances. They were then asked which verbs appeared to be "more frequent" (although this was likely difficult to manage with a large volume of concordances). In the next activity, students were guided to use wildcards firstly to replace the verb in the query term 'the data suggest that', noting the verbs that could fill that slot, before secondly adding a wildcard to the query term 'calculate*', which would provide some data as to the different forms of the lemma. Students were then directed to query the term 'calculate' in the both the professional and learner corpus, before being asked "what do the results tell you?". Lastly, students consulted both corpora for the query term 'undoubtedly', and were asked "what they noticed about the differences" based on what they could derive from reading the concordances and looking at the frequency information.

Regarding the language case tasks themselves, 'Language Case 1' (Figure 5.2) was introduced in lesson 3 of the materials, focusing on the appropriate use of tenses when writing a literature review. These activities were intended to be conducted out-of-class, before students met with their tutors and peers the next week to discuss their findings.

This activity is framed in a similar manner to the 'problem-based learning' pedagogical approach that the dental students were used to experiencing in their disciplinary content courses. The activity begins with a 2-part "problem statement", outlining the issue Jeff is experiencing, before students were asked to "make some searches" within the professional and learner corpora using the corpus platform. Students should "select some examples" from the concordances, then "explain the linguistic findings" to their peers and tutors in class the following week. The "trigger

CAES9350 *Academic English for Dentistry* Semester 2, 2016–2017

Summary of Language Problem 1: Making the Right Choice

Author: Dr. Lisa Cheung

Session 4: 6 February 2017

Language Problem Statement

Part 1

Jeff is a BDSV student. He is writing a research report for his project. He remembered his English teacher taught in class that different tenses could be used in writing the Literature Review, but he couldn't figure out the rationale for tense choice. He just felt he would use the simple past tense ...

Part 2

Jeff has been reading some research papers. He found different tense uses in the Literature Review. He got puzzled, "What tense shall I use then?"

Product

Make some searches on the *Dentistry Corpus Search Site* (search the professional and learner corpora).
Select some examples from your searches.
Explain the linguistic findings to your teacher/group members.

Anticipated Learning Issues

Choice of tenses in writing the Literature Review
Choice of verbs in citing sources

Trigger Questions

1. Why did Jeff think he should use the simple past tense in writing the Literature Review?
2. Why did the teacher say in class that different tenses could be used in writing the Literature Review?
3. Is it possible to use more than one tense in the Literature Review? What is the principle that governs Jeff's choice?
4. Which tense is most frequently used in the Literature Review in Dentistry? Can you find some examples from your corpus search?
5. Which reporting verbs are com only used in Dentistry? Can you find some examples from your corpus search?

Learning Resource for Students

Dentistry Corpus Search Site (via HKU Moodle)

Figure 5.2 Language Case 1: 'Making the right choice'

questions" were intended to help students complete the main activity by offering additional starting points from which to conduct corpus queries, such as asking students to determine "Which tense is most frequently used in the literature review?"

Language Case 2 (Figure 5.3) uses the same approach to get students to query hedges and boosters in both professional and learner corpora. Students could attempt to answer trigger questions 4 and 5 shown in the figure by querying these devices from a list provided in a previous unit. They would then meet with the disciplinary tutors and their peers to discuss their findings the following week.

CAES9350 *Academic English for Dentistry* Semester 2, 2016–2017

Summary of Language Problem 2: To hedge or not to hedge **Session 8: 20 March 2017**	**Author: Dr. Lisa Cheung**
Language Problem Statement Amy is a BDSV student. Last week she wrote up the Discussion section of her Community Health Project report. Her English teacher assessed her written work, and wrote some comments (see the next page). Amy was surprised to see that some sentences were underlined with the comment *"Be cautious in making claims. Hedge the sentence!"* She got puzzled, "Why hedging?" ... **Product** Make some searches on the *Dentistry Corpus Search Site* (search the professio nal and learner corpora). Select some examples from your searches. Explain the linguistic findings to your teacher/group members.	**Anticipated Learning Issues** Making reasonable claims Use of hedges and boosters **Trigger Questions** 1. Why did Amy's teacher underline some sentences in Amy's work. and ask her to *"be cautious in making claims"*? What do you think the problems are with these sentences? 2. Why did the teacher want Amy to 'hedge' these sentences? What is a hedge? What is a booster? 3. Can you suggest some possible reasons governing the use of hedges and boosters in making claims? 4. Which hedges are most frequently used in making claims in Dentistry? Can you find some examples from your corpus search? 5. Which boosters are most frequently used in making claims in Dentistry? Can you find some examples from your corpus search? **Learning Resource for Students** *Dentistry Corpus Search Site (via HKU Moodle)*

Figure 5.3 Language Case 2: 'To Hedge or Not to Hedge'

It should be clear to the reader that despite our best intentions, we were asking a lot of the ED students to complete these activities. The activities relied on students being able to easily manipulate the concordance output, a task made increasingly difficult the more concordances appeared. Despite "concordancing tools [being] the key instruments for analysing corpora" (Gavioli, 2005: p. 11), the reliance on concordance output alone made answering a number of the trigger questions a laborious task, especially if more than one page of concordance output was produced. It must also be said here that producing concordance output was quite slow under this version of the corpus platform. Wildcard queries could take up to 30 seconds to be displayed, especially if multiple users were conducting queries simultaneously. The Language Case' activities, despite being framed in a way that the dentistry students were used to when taking their disciplinary content courses, likely provided insufficient scaffolding for students in determining *what* and *how* to query the corpus when resolving the issues outlined in each activity, leaving interpretations and concluding analysis entirely up to the students. This is made even more serious given the very short (2 hour) training session provided, of which only the second hour was spent querying the corpus. This was likely insufficient for students to be fully aware of the functionality of the corpus platform under our supervision before they were left with no further guidance upon completion of the training session. This may have been insufficient in getting students to understand and acquire the basic techniques for interpreting concordance lines in an effective manner, such as grouping concordance lines to test a language hypothesis (Sinclair, 1999). This likely demotivated students in using the corpus platform to resolve their language issues.

These difficulties were eventually reflected in student course and teaching evaluations. Upon completion of this first run of the ED course, students' course effectiveness evaluations reached a disappointing 55.8 out of 100 points. An accompanying Course Quality Questionnaire (CQQ) pressed the matter further, garnering an 88.2% response rate. While students were generally satisfied that they had met the learning outcomes of "*Deploying strategies for research report writing and apply these when writing different sections of a report*" (67.2% satisfied) and "*Using appropriate language to present research findings based on relevant review of literature, research methods, data collection, and recommendations*" (71.1% satisfied), students were much less enthusiastic about the dentistry corpus resources built into the course. Students' response to the item "*The eLearning resources (e.g. Out-of-class Learning Modules on the Moodle site, Dentistry Corpus Search) have provided useful support for self-directed learning*" garnered only a 42.8% satisfaction rate, clearly well below expectation. Students also complained that the activities were not pitched at the right level (56.7% satisfied) and that the tasks were not appropriate for a fifth-year Dentistry undergraduate ED course (53.9% satisfied). Qualitative comments focusing on the corpus activities revealed the following:

> Corpus: This is an interesting tool that I would like to learn, but the technology and quality of the corpus hinder my learning
>
> [The] Corpus is not working. The tasks on corpus could be redesigned, and the instruction was unclear
>
> Corpus: Too slow to process in class, and search results were little [sic] especially for the learner corpus

These evaluations were administered by the university centrally. To focus more specifically on the DDL aspect of the course, we modified a DDL-specific post-course questionnaire published originally in Yoon and Hirvela (2004). This questionnaire is divided into sections related to the benefits of using the corpus, the difficulties encountered, usage of corpora for writing beyond the course, and a section we added focusing on disciplinary issues. Only 16 students completed the questionnaire, so we interpret the results with caution.

Regarding the benefits of the DDL provision (Table 5.1), while students generally agreed that searching the corpus for concordances was easy to learn and that they felt confident in using the platform, they tended to disagree that the corpus was more helpful than dictionaries, doubted its effectiveness for learning disciplinary vocabulary and grammar, and disagreed that it improved their academic writing.

Table 5.1 Benefits of the DDL provision in ED's first iteration

Statement	Strongly disagree	Disagree	Somewhat agree	Agree	Strongly agree
1. The corpus searching technique was easy to learn	0(0.0%)	1(6.3%)	6(37.5%)	7(43.8%)	2(12.5%)
2. I feel confident in answering questions about my writing using a corpus	0(0.0%)	2(12.5%)	9(56.3%)	4(25.0%)	1(6.3%)
3. The corpus is more helpful than a dictionary for my English writing	2(12.5%)	6(37.5%)	5(31.3%)	3(18.8%)	0(0.0%)
4. Using the corpus is helpful for learning the meaning of disciplinary vocabulary	0(0.0%)	7(43.8%)	6(37.5%)	3(18.8%)	0(0.0%)
5. Using the corpus is helpful for learning the usage of disciplinary vocabulary	0(0.0%)	5(31.3%)	6(37.5%)	5(31.3%)	0(0.0%)
6. Using the corpus is helpful for the usage of phrases	0(0.0%)	5(31.3%)	6(37.5%)	5(31.3%)	0(0.0%)
7. Using the corpus is helpful for learning grammar	1(6.3%)	6(37.5%)	7(43.8%)	2(12.5%)	0(0.0%)
8. Using the corpus improved my English writing skill	2(12.5%)	6(37.5%)	4(25.0%)	3(18.8%)	0(0.0%)
9. Using the corpus improved my academic writing ability, especially research report writing	1(6.3%)	5(31.3%)	6(37.5%)	4(25.0%)	0(0.0%)

The results regarding perceived difficulty in using the corpus are more encouraging (Table 5.2), with most students disagreeing with each of the questions for this section of the questionnaire. However, as the polarity of each question in this section is negative while the polarity of questions in other sections of the questionnaire are positive, we cannot avoid the possibility that students may have answered these questions incorrectly if they were completing the questionnaire in a hurry.

Table 5.2 Students' perceived difficulties in using the corpus platform

Statement	Strongly disagree	Disagree	Somewhat agree	Agree	Strongly agree
10. I have some difficulty in using the corpus due to time and effort spent analyzing the data	1(6.3%)	7(43.8%)	5(31.3%)	2(12.5%)	1(6.3%)
11. I have some difficulty in using the corpus due to unfamiliar vocabulary on concordance output	2(12.5%)	6(37.5%)	5(31.3%)	3(18.8%)	0(0.0%)
12. I have some difficulty in using the corpus due to cut-off sentences in the concordance output	2(12.5%)	7(43.8%)	5(31.3%)	2(12.5%)	0(0.0%)
13. I have some difficulty in using the corpus due to too many sentences in concordance output	2(12.5%)	7(43.8%)	4(25.0%)	3(18.8%)	0(0.0%)
14. I have some difficulty in using the corpus due to the limited number of sentences in concordance output	4(25.0%)	6(37.5%)	3(18.8%)	3(18.8%)	0(0.0%)
15. I have some difficulty in analyzing concordance output	2(12.5%)	5(31.3%)	5(31.3%)	4(25.0%)	0(0.0%)
16. I have some difficulty understanding the teacher's feedback to correct my writing	4(25.0%)	6(37.5%)	4(25.0%)	2(12.5%)	0(0.0%)
17. I have some difficulty converting the teacher's feedback into corpus queries	2(12.5%)	8(50.0%)	4(25.0%)	1(6.3%)	1(6.3%)
18. I have some difficulty correcting errors in my writing using the corpus outside class	2(12.5%)	7(43.8%)	4(25.0%)	3(18.8%)	0(0.0%)
19. I have some difficulty in performing the search technique	2(12.5%)	9(56.3%)	3(18.8%)	2(12.5%)	0(0.0%)
20. The real texts in the corpus are too difficult to understand	2(12.5%)	11(68.8%)	1(6.3%)	2(12.5%)	0(0.0%)

The results in Table 5.3 are more disappointing, with students apparently unwilling to use the corpus under their own initiative, most lamenting its usefulness, and with most unwilling to want to use the corpus again. The poor results overall for this first iteration of the ED course were incredibly disappointing, with most students claiming the corpus was not a useful resource for English writing, and that using the corpus had not improved their writing of the dentistry register, although they did suggest that a disciplinary corpus was still more useful than a general corpus. As with the other aspects of the ED course during this iteration, it is also likely that students see little point in consulting a corpus solely for completing ED activities in class. Gavioli (2005: p. 19), citing Widdowson (1998) in his critique of corpus-based pedagogy, suggests that it is not enough to simply expose students to passages from a specialised corpus, as this does not guarantee that they will "authenticate" the language within their disciplinary context. Rather, it was quickly determined that the corpus activities and platform, as well as the entire ED provision itself, would be of much greater benefit if they were actually contextualised within the main disciplinary content and assessments of the dentistry degree, rather than being located at the periphery. This necessitated a rethink of the entire ED corpus provision, as described in the next section.

Table 5.3 Students' responses regarding corpora and writing/disciplinary use

Statement	Strongly disagree	Disagree	Somewhat agree	Agree	Strongly agree
21. I often use the corpus by my own choice	7(43.8%)	5(31.3%)	4(25.0%)	0(0.0%)	0(0.0%)
22. I understand the purpose of using the corpus in this course	0(0.0%)	1(6.3%)	8(50.0%)	6(37.5%)	1(6.3%)
23. I want to use the corpus in my next English writing course	1(6.3%)	7(43.8%)	6(37.5%)	2(12.5%)	0(0.0%)
24. When I have a problem in my English writing, I search for help in the corpus	3(18.8%)	7(43.8%)	5(31.3%)	1(6.3%)	0(0.0%)
25. When I search for information in the corpus, I usually get the information that I need	2(12.5%)	6(37.5%)	7(43.8%)	1(6.3%)	0(0.0%)
26. I use the corpus when writing papers for other courses too	6(37.5%)	8(50.0%)	2(12.5%)	0(0.0%)	0(0.0%)
27. As I have learned more about the corpus I have come to like them more	3(18.8%)	5(31.3%)	8(50.0%)	0(0.0%)	0(0.0%)
28. I will use the corpus for my English writing in the future	3(18.8%)	6(37.5%)	6(37.5%)	1(6.3%)	0(0.0%)
29. Learning about the corpus has increased my confidence about writing in English	3(18.8%)	8(50.0%)	4(25.0%)	1(6.3%)	0(0.0%)
30. Overall, the corpus is a very useful resource for my English writing	2(12.5%)	6(37.5%)	7(43.8%)	1(6.3%)	0(0.0%)
----------	----------	----------	----------	----------	----------
31. A dentistry-specific corpus is more useful than a general corpus	1(6.3%)	1(6.3%)	7(43.8%)	5(31.3%)	2(12.5%)
32. I learned vocabulary specific to dentistry using the corpus	0(0.0%)	5(31.3%)	8(50.0%)	3(18.8%)	0(0.0%)
33. I am better at writing in a dentistry register after using the corpus	0(0.0%)	5(31.3%)	9(56.3%)	2(12.5%)	0(0.0%)

5.5 Trying again: A new corpus platform

To facilitate further ED corpus pedagogy, we utilised a corpus platform developed as part of a project to introduce DDL into post-graduate disciplinary thesis writing, headed by Dr. Lillian Wong and the first author of this volume as described in Crosthwaite, Wong and Cheung (2019), modifying the interface and corpus used for dentistry ED. We worked alongside computer programmers to develop a novel online corpus query platform that would allow students to investigate the professional and learner corpora of CHP reports in much more detail and with a wider array of entry points into the corpus data. As previous iterations of the online platform only allowed for concordances to be produced, this new platform needed to incorporate a greater range of corpus query functions and data visualisation procedures so as to drastically improve the usability of the online platform for novice users. In addition, we also incorporated a range of learner tracking analytics into the system (see Chapter 6). This would also allow us to meaningfully track the query patterns and usage histories of users with a view to further improving the corpus platform and related activities in future iterations of the ESAP course. A screenshot of the platform's new front end is shown in Figure 5.4.

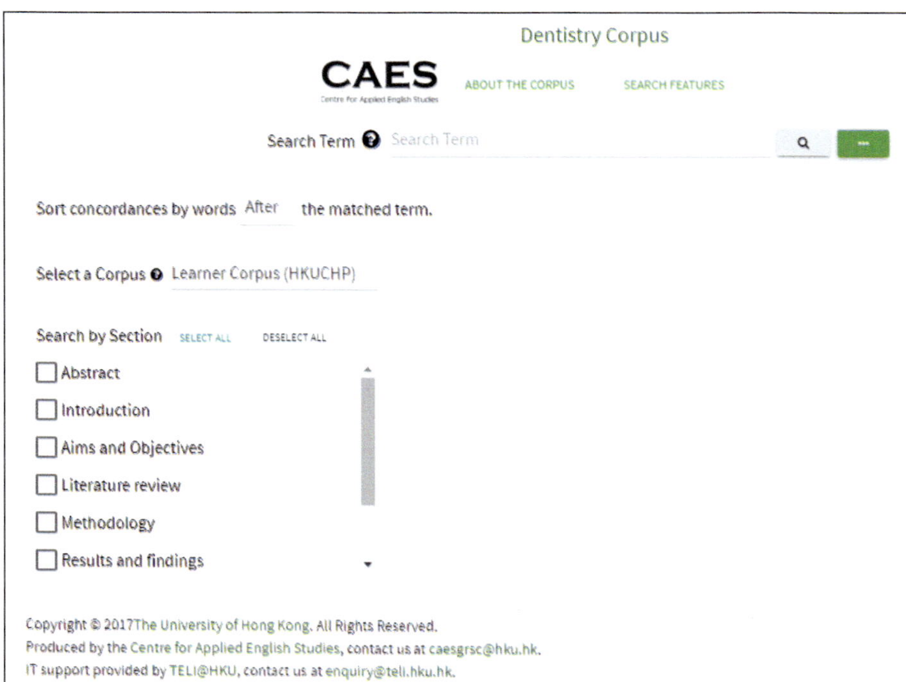

Figure 5.4 Corpus query platform user interface main menu

Here, users can enter their query syntax into the 'search term' bar, and select to have the resulting concordances sorted to the left or right of the query term. They also have the option to conduct their query within the professional or learner CHP corpora. For the learner corpus, students can filter the returned hits by section, although at the time of writing this functionality was not available for the professional corpus. Users can perform single word or multi-word searches as well as searches including wildcards attached to or replacing words or phrases (e.g. "dent*" would display results including "dental", "dentistry", "dentalgia"). Users can also search via POS tags, or combine these with wildcards (e.g. 'was *_v' would bring up concordances for passive constructions. Supported tags include n = noun, v = verb, adj = adjective, adv = adverb, pp = preposition, cc = conjunction and md = modal. Figure 5.5 shows part of the concordance display for the term 'tooth' within the professional corpus.

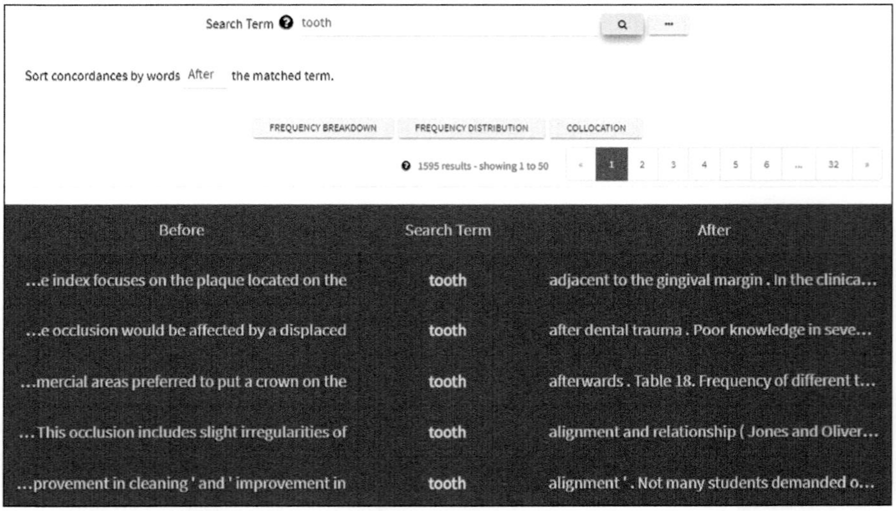

Figure 5.5 Concordance sample for 'tooth' in the professional corpus

Three additional functions were implemented for this interface. *Frequency breakdown* provides a bar chart with the most frequent hits for the query, with Figure 5.6 showing the results for the query 'tooth *'.

The *frequency distribution* function can be used to show the distribution of a given search by section (Figure 5.7), here showing results for the term 'data' in the learner corpus.

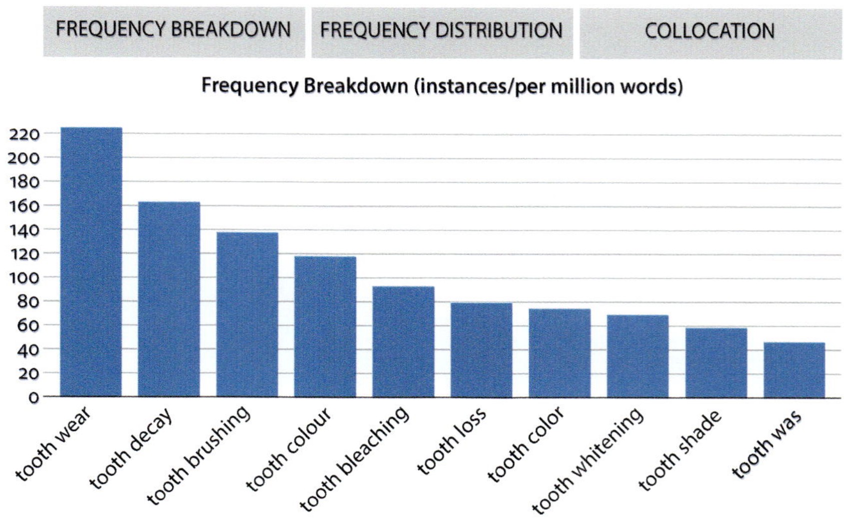

Figure 5.6 Results for the 'Frequency Breakdown' function for the query 'tooth *'

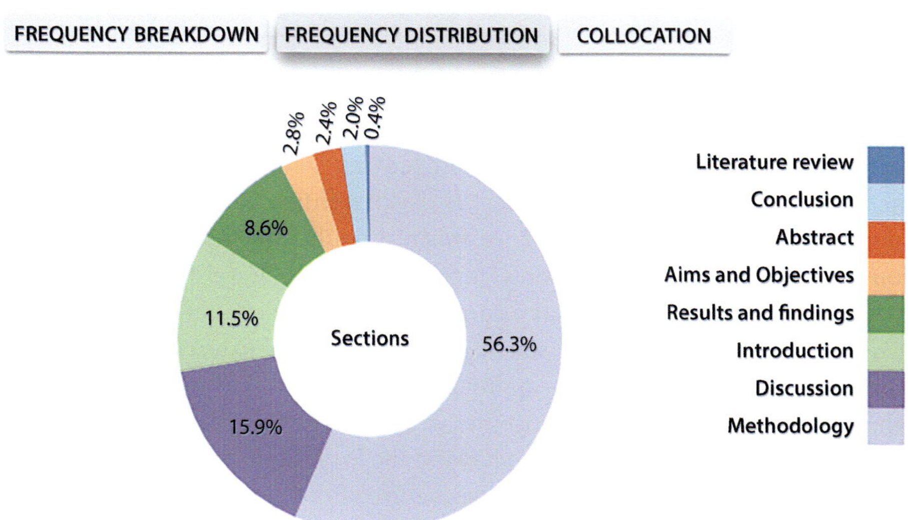

Figure 5.7 'Frequency Distribution' function by section in the learner corpus

Finally, *collocation* presents a visual display of collocates, with the search term located in the centre, and collocations one word to the **left/right** of the query term shown on the left-hand / right-hand side of the centre term respectively (Figure 5.8). Positioning to the left/right is determined by frequency of occurrence in the corpus, with more frequent items closer to the centre and shown in orange, with less frequent items more on the periphery and displayed in green. Figure 5.8 shows the results of this function for the query term 'were'.

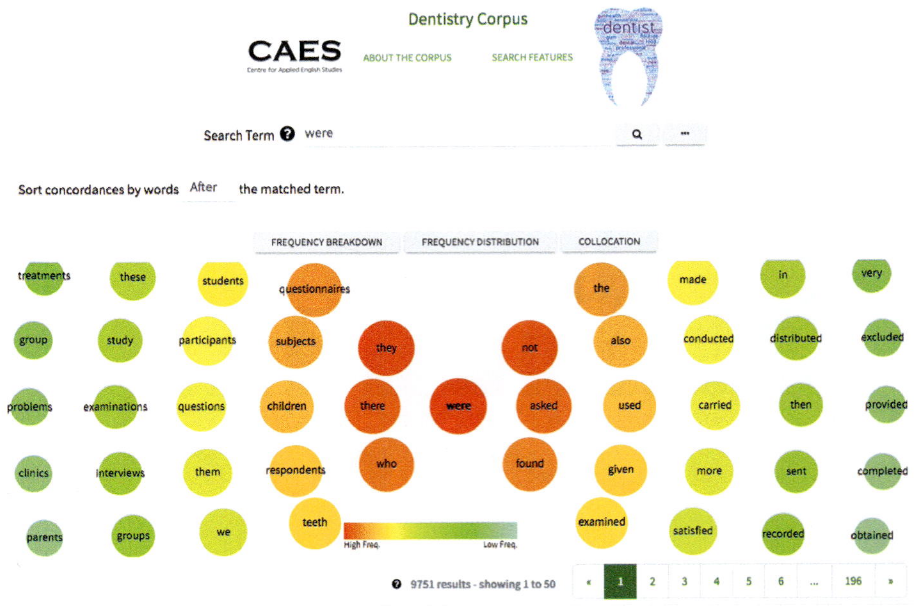

Figure 5.8 Sample results for 'were' using the 'collocation' function in the learner corpus

Together, the new functionality and visual presentation of the corpus platform was a massive improvement on previous practice, and allowed for much greater variety and flexibility in the kind of accompanying DDL activities we planned to incorporate into the ED study materials. By presenting students with multiple sources of information in this way, we are creating the necessary conditions for a constructivist approach to DDL and language learning (Flowerdew, 2015), in that "the more possible starting points a corpus offers for exploitation, the more likely it is there exists an appropriate starting point for a specific learner" (Widmann, Kohn & Ziai, 2011: p. 168). This approach is seen in the work of Charles (2015), who incorporates concordances together with tools to derive word lists, collocates and concordance plots (i.e. images showing the location of query hits within the whole text or corpus). The highly visual nature of the data also works to ensure those with more visual learning styles can engage with DDL, a consideration again noted in Flowerdew (2015) as important for learning.

5.6 Corpus tasks

Designing DDL tasks involving direct, hand-on use of corpora for the purposes of writing instruction is not an easy task. Ädel (2010) outlines seven challenges facing the budding DDL task designer, including lack of corpus availability; the "corpus as a maze" of linguistic information, which risks students "drowning in data" (p. 45); difficulty of interpreting and evaluating corpus data; the dangers of decontextualized data; and a focus on surface form. There are also challenges in designing DDL tasks within disciplinary writing contexts, including the differing needs of individual learners for language-focused tasks (Römer, 2011), the relative need for discipline-specificity in light of cross-departmental EGAP/ESAP provision, and the relative teacher vs. student-focused approach to learning in the classroom (Anthony, 2016). Our goal was to develop DDL materials that drew on the analyses of previous chapters, promoted 'writing-to-learn', and overcome the learner- and corpus-related challenges outlined in the literature. Meeting some of these challenges was easier than others – availability of the corpus was now a non-issue, the context of the data was clear to students, and the needs of the learners were (comparatively speaking at least) homogenous for this cohort of learners within our narrow disciplinary context. The remaining challenges for us involved guiding students to avoid "drowning in detail" and to be able to interpret and evaluate corpus data with ease. The remainder of this chapter describes how we met these challenges in more detail.

In total, seven individual DDL activities (titled "corpus tasks" in the Course Booklet), involving multiple stages to completion, were developed for in-class use, with a range of other activities designed for out-of-class use. Much of the content for these tasks is based around the findings from Chapters 2 to 4, as well as on additional content related to composition already included in previous versions of the course materials. Other course materials feature a series of 'top-down' activities focusing on larger segments of texts and the move structure of key sections of the research report. Many of the exemplars in these segments were sourced from our disciplinary corpus, following similar provision in Charles (2007), Cortes (2007), and Tribble and Wingate (2013). Some activities focused primarily on bottom-up language features in the form of gap-fills or multiple-choice questions, and it is these tasks that were prime targets for revision into tasks involving the corpus. The combination of the top-down and bottom-up tasks make for "the best of both worlds" (Charles, 2014: p. 299) in that "discipline-specific corpora can be exploited for bottom-up explorations of how genre, as a form of social action, enables and constrains linguistic choices, as well as for top-down DDL to engage students in a critical analysis of the discourse of their target disciplinary communities" (Cotos, Link & Huffman, 2017: p. 106).

As in Aston (1995) and Hafner and Candlin (2007), the activities were integrated into the course materials alongside other pre-existing non-corpus-based tasks. Activities were based around a particular problem or situation that the students would encounter as novice writers, so as to maintain the 'authenticity' of any associated corpus use. The sequencing of the tasks and the detailed rubrics provided also served as an indirect method of training students in the use of the corpus platform and its associated functions, rather than devoting extensive class time to direct training in corpus queries. Our approach therefore follows Perez-Parades et al. (2011), who distinguish *guided* corpus consultation tasks involving carefully selected specific language features and corpus functions for investigation, to relatively 'unguided' tasks where students could select their own language features for analysis depending on their discipline Perez-Parades et al.'s (2011) study suggested that the guided condition was preferable to the unguided condition, although in most cases this guidance comes from explicit teacher-led training prior to corpus consultation. Our approach did not require lengthy explicit training or guidance in the corpus functions prior to taking on the corpus tasks embedded in the course materials. Rather, the goal was to ensure that the scaffolding required for students to (a) complete the tasks and (b) become proficient in using the corpus was embedded in the tasks themselves, through their sequencing, instructional rubrics, open-ended questions, use of exemplar queries and results prior to corpus use, and the incorporation of a collaborative aspect to certain tasks. We took this cue from Molés-Cases and Oster (2015), who successfully incorporated DDL into the curriculum for translation students in the form of 'webquests' where students consulted online resources to complete open-ended tasks requiring collaboration and critical thinking. Charles (2015: p. 150) also suggests that such collaboration "fosters richer understandings and insights" while also being "an important step for students in their on-going attempt to be full members of their field". Another aim was for our activities to follow, as much as possible, Carter and McCarthy's (1995) "3 Is", namely:

1. Illustration (looking at data)
2. Interaction (discussion and sharing observations and opinions)
3. Induction (making one's own rule for a particular feature).

The sequence is intended to promote the necessary conditions for DDL to promote 'noticing', which is required for any focus on form to be effective (Flowerdew, 2015).

The first corpus task is introduced in the second unit of the course booklet, which focuses on the structural moves and language features of the introduction section within a scientific research report. This includes top-down awareness-raising activities on the typical move structures in the introduction (e.g. Swales, 1990) such as identifying a research topic, reviewing current knowledge on the topic, identifying a gap in the current knowledge on the topic, and identifying the sub topics / research questions for their own investigations. The task also focuses on the verb tenses typically used within the introduction section, where high frequencies of present tense forms are found, with low frequencies of past tense forms. Corpus task 1 (Figure 5.9) explores the circumstances in which academic writers can refer to themselves directly in the introduction / aims and objectives sections of a scientific research report, with data discussed in Chapter 3 (see also Crosthwaite, Cheung & Jiang, 2017) showing that novice dentistry CHP writers are significantly more likely to insert themselves into their texts as compared with professional writers.

Corpus task

Corpus Task 1: Referring to yourself in the Introduction
Using the Learner Corpus, search for 'My', remembering to select the 'Introduction' and "Aims and Objectives' sections in the search menu.

1. Is '**My**' commonly used in Community Health Project report writing?
2. What words are usually found after '**My**' (click 'collocation', and look for words that occur after '**My**')
3. Repeat 1–2 for '**Our**' – what do you notice?
4. Repeat 1–2 for '**We**' – what do you notice?
5. Based on 1–4, discuss with a partner the following: Under what circumstances can we refer to ourselves directly in the Introductions / Aims and Objectives of the CHP reports?

Figure 5.9 Corpus task 1

Regarding the answer to question 1 in Figure 5.9, querying 'my' in the learner corpus results in a frequency count of 4.78 hits per million words, with just 4 actual hits. Students are then instructed in class that this would be a very low frequency result within this corpus, and were informed that by implication, 'my' is unlikely to be used in CHP report introductions or aims and objectives sections. Figure 5.10 shows the results retrieved via using the *collocation* function for the second question in Figure 5.10.

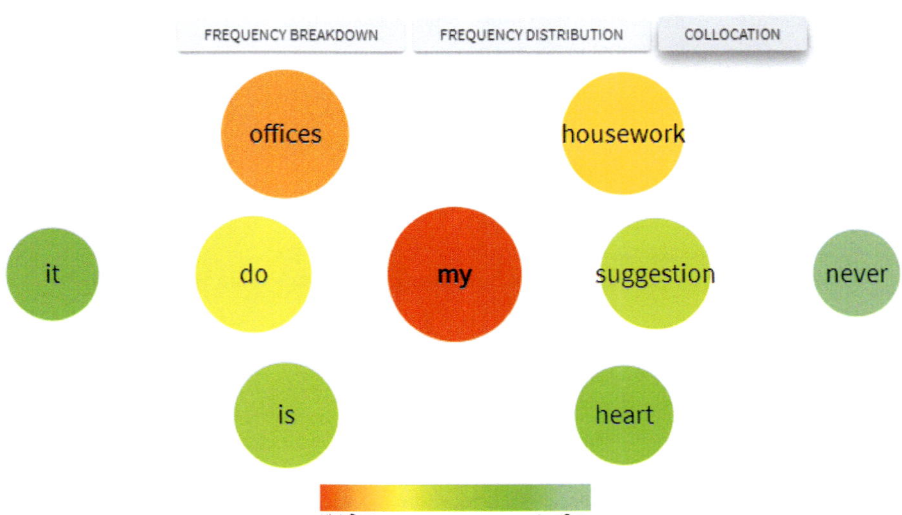

Figure 5.10 Collocation results for 'my' in the learner corpus

The results shown here, including 'housework', 'suggestion', and 'heart', are derived from only 4 hits each, and students are made aware that the low frequency colour coding each result is given is further evidence that they are potentially unreliable collocates. Regarding the comparison with 'our', which has a frequency of 385.77 hits per million words with 323 raw hits in the corpus, students are informed that this is a relatively high frequency of occurrence when compared with 'my'. Following discussion of these results with their peers, the intention is for students to realise that the data now strongly suggests that (a) students may refer to themselves in the introduction and aims and objectives sections, and (b) if they do wish to refer to themselves in academic writing, they should use the first-person plural and plural possessive.

The second corpus task (Figure 5.10) focuses on the use of reporting verbs used for reviewing current knowledge on an academic topic in the literature review section of the thesis. This activity introduces the wildcard feature of the corpus query platform to students for the first time, allowing them to use this feature to explore variants of a common reporting verb construction. The selection of this particular construction for analysis was based on our finding from our MDA in Chapter 2 under the dimension *involved vs. informational discourse,* which showed that the use of the perfect construction (as a more 'involved' form of discourse)

Corpus task

Corpus Task 2: Verbs for reviewing current knowledge on a topic
Using the Learner Corpus, enter the phrase 'Studies have * that', then click 'frequency breakdown' (**select all sections in the corpus**).

1. List 4 verbs that are commonly used in place of the wildcard (*) in the search phrase 'studies have * that'.
   a. ____________________
   b. ____________________
   c. ____________________
   d. ____________________
   From this list, rank them in terms of how strong the author's claim is about that research.
2. Click on the chart column for 'studies have shown that'. Write 3 sentences that begin with 'studies have shown that' from those results.
   a. Studies have shown that ______________________________
   b. Studies have shown that ______________________________
   c. Studies have shown that ______________________________
3. Replace 'studies' with a wildcard * ('* have shown that). List 4 variants of 'studies' in this construction.
   a. ______________________________ have shown that
   b. ______________________________ have shown that
   c. ______________________________ have shown that
   d. ______________________________ have shown that

Figure 5.11 Corpus task 2

was common when describing others' previous findings in the literature review section of dental research reports. The activity uses Sinclair's (1991) idiom principle as its basis, taking our pre-constructed word combination 'studies have shown that', and getting students to explore the corpus for alternatives. Here, students can realise that rather than a fixed 'idiomatic' expression, the corpus data points to this construction as being an 'open choice' construction, where variance (after 'that') may be likely to occur as long as the other elements remain largely the same. The resultant concordances and frequency information derived from their corpus queries provide further information as to which constructions are a) potentially grammatical; and b) used in disciplinary writing. Potential answers to question 1 in Figure 5.11 include 'suggested', 'reported' and 'demonstrated', while students were

Corpus task

Corpus Task 3: More on writing the Literature Review
Use the Professional Corpus to complete the following activities.
Present perfect tense

1. Enter the term 'research has *'. Click 'frequency breakdown'. Which verbs are shown in the chart? What tense are they in?
2. Click on the chart column for one of the verbs shown in 1). Write 5 sentences using that verb.
   a. Research has ______________________________
   b. Research has ______________________________
   c. Research has ______________________________
   d. Research has ______________________________
   e. Research has ______________________________

Signal the literature gap
Now, use the Learner Corpus to complete the following activities (**ensure that Introduction, and Aims and Objectives sections are checked for each question**).

1. Enter 'few' into the search bar. Write down 5 sentences containing 'few' that appear to signal a 'gap' in the literature
   a. ______________ few ______________________
   b. ______________ few ______________________
   c. ______________ few ______________________

   Click 'collocation'. Which noun might be used together with 'few' to signal a gap in the literature?
   Click 'studies' and click 'frequency distribution'. Is the expression 'few studies' more likely to occur in the *introduction*, or *aims and objectives* sections?
   Now, repeat (1) to (3) for the word 'little' (except 'studies' will not be the answer for step 2). What do you notice about the differences in the way 'few' and 'little' are used to signal the research gap?
   Discuss with a partner about when and why you might use 'few' and 'little' to signal a 'gap' in the literature.

Figure 5.12 Corpus task 3

free to add their own examples for question 2 from the resultant concordances. Potential answers for question 3 include 'countries', 'results' and 'siblings'.

The first section of corpus task 3 (see Figure 5.12) again involves the use of the perfect (albeit this time using the professional corpus), while the second section focuses on how writers can signal a 'gap' in the literature through the use of 'few' and 'little'. For the second section of the corpus task involving the learner corpus, searching for 'few' and consulting the concordances provides some clue as to the target expression for question 1 (Figure 5.13), while for the second question, 'studies', 'attempts', and 'articles' are potential answers, with 'studies' shown as the more frequent collocate (Figure 5.14). Students can then determine whether the 'gap' should be added to the introduction or aims and objectives sections of the research report by consulting the distribution of 'few studies' in both sections by answering the third question (Figure 5.15).

...neral population1-5. There have been only a	few	studies about the oral hygiene status of priso...
...nts had the condition (Schuurs et al. , 1995).	Few	studies have been carried out in countries ot...
...hod of evaluating CDS has yet to be resolved.	Few	studies have examined differences in self-rep...
...e of asthma among children, there have been	few	studies investigating the correlation between...
...ut oral health status behind bars. Among the	few	studies that exist; it has been suggested that ...
...eats to the public.3 However, there are only a	few	studies to measure how the media is influenc...
...ortant role in a successful practice. Though a	few	textbooks on dental practice management ar...

Figure 5.13 Sample concordance lines for 'few' in the learner corpus

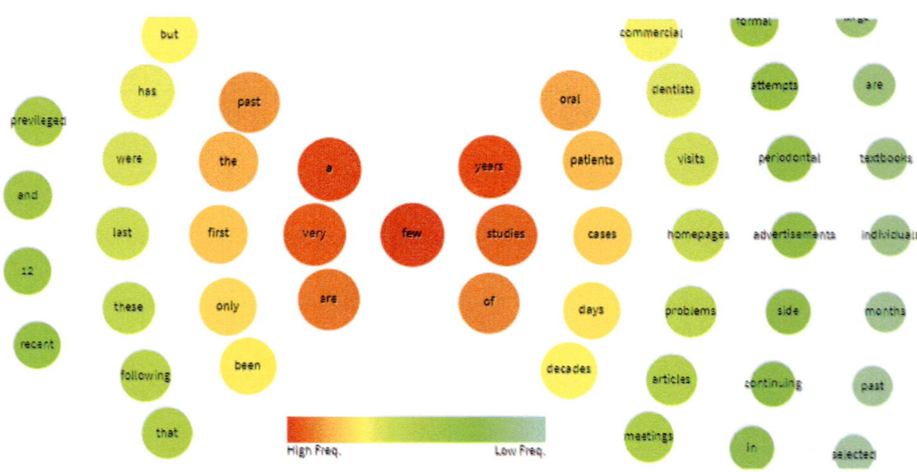

Figure 5.14 Collocates of 'few' in the learner corpus

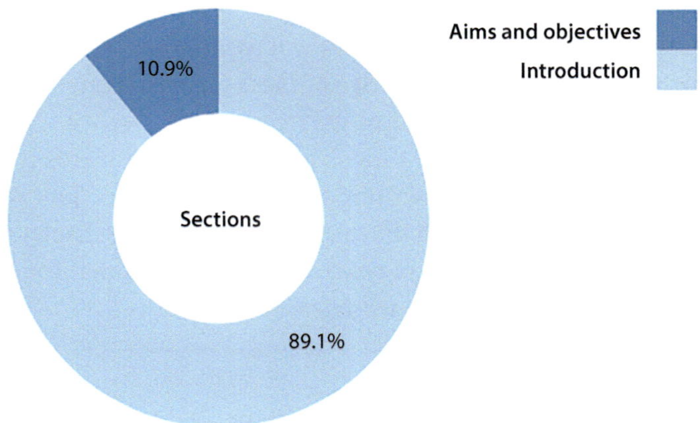

Figure 5.15 Distribution of 'few studies' by section in the learner corpus

While these features were not highlighted in Chapters 2 to 4, this corpus activity is used to prepare students for the top-down task in Figure 5.16, requiring students to write a paragraph signalling a 'gap' in previous research when writing the introduction to a research paper.

Long-term implant survival and success: a 10–16-year follow-up of non-submerged dental implants

Pierre Simonis, Thomas Dufour and Henri Tenenbaum

Introduction

A great number of studies have analysed the survival of oral implants, mostly for up to 5 years. Few studies have followed up implants over the long term. The survival of dental implants before loading is very high. An initial loss of 2–3% in all implants is followed by another 2–3% loss over an observation period of 5 years for implants supporting fixed partial dentures (FPDs). In the overdenture treatment, 45% of the implants are lost within the same 5-year period (Holm-Pedersen et al. 2007). Ten-year results were only reported in a few studies (Leonhardt et al. 2002; Karoussis et al. 2003, 2004; Roos-Jansaker et al. 2006a, 2006b, 2006c). When the longevity of fixed prosthesis was addressed, systematic reviews showed a survival rate of 96.5% after 5 years for single tooth replacement, 95.4% for implant–implant fixed bridgework and 90.1% for implant–tooth reconstruction (Lang et al. 2004; Pjetursson et al. 2004a, 2004b; Bragger et al. 2005; Jung et al. 2008). Nevertheless, the notions of survival and success are often used in a confusing manner, although precise definitions are available (Albrektsson et al. 1986; Smith & Zarb 1989).

____

____

____

____

____

Figure 5.16 Signalling the research gap

Having already explored the function and usage of 'few' and 'little' in the preceding corpus task, the expectation is that students will use this next activity as an opportunity to test their new-found knowledge of these forms to complete this crucial 'move' of a research article introduction.

Corpus task 4 (see Figure 5.17) involves the use of wildcards to investigate the typical verb tenses used when writing the methodology section. A number of these verbs have been selected from the case report analysis in Chapter 4, including 'correct' and 'advocate' from the list of *positive verbs*, 'affect' from the *modify/change* semantic field, and 'notice' from the *sensory* semantic field.

Corpus task

Corpus task 4: Using wildcards to learn about verb forms

Search the **Learner Corpus** to complete the following activities (**ensure the Methodology section is checked**).

A. Use the wildcard * immediately after a word's base form as well as the frequency breakdown function to get an idea about which tense to use when using these verbs to write the methodology section (e.g. use*). Write the different forms of the verb that appear in the results (Note that some of these verbs will be in the passive voice, requiring the addition of the correct 'be' verb).

1. Test ____________________
2. Use ____________________
3. Correct ____________________
4. Obtain ____________________
5. Advocate ____________________
6. Affect ____________________
7. Notice ____________________
8. Investigate ____________________

B. Use the results above to decide which tense is typically used when writing the methodology section

Figure 5.17 Corpus task 4

Students querying 'use*' then selecting the *frequency breakdown* function will be able to see that the past tense form of the lemma 'use' is much more frequently used than the present tense form (Figure 5.18), as is the case for the rest of the target verbs in questions 1–8. This information can then be used to answer the question shown in section B of the task.

While not requiring students to use the corpus itself, corpus task 5-1 focuses on writing the abstract of the research report, and is based on the MDA conducted on the professional *Community Dental Health* corpus in Chapter 3. The task asks students to label the highlighted sections in a sample abstract taken from one of

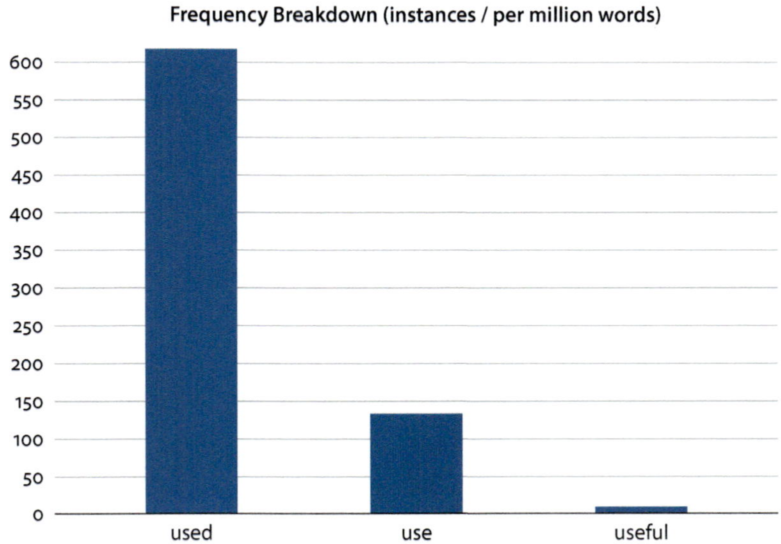

Figure 5.18 Words beginning with 'use' in the methodology section in the learner corpus

the papers in the professional corpus, with each excerpt selected as an exemplar of the linguistic features that characterise each of the five dimensions derived from the MDA. Present tense verbs were an 'informative' feature of Dimension 1 (narrative vs. informative), used by professional writers to communicate their findings as facts. Nouns and nominalisations were an 'objective' feature of Dimension 2 (persuasive vs. objective) with student texts more likely to contain possibility modals, infinitives and associated base form verbs. Evaluative adjectives, passive voice constructions, and numbers/numerical conversions were each key linguistic features of Dimensions 3 (tentative vs. authoritative), Dimension 4 (active vs. passive), and Dimension 5 (animate vs. inanimate) respectively. Upon completion of the labelling task, students then match these language forms to their associated function in abstract writing. The suggested answers are shown in red font in Figure 5.19.

Corpus task

Corpus task 5–1: The dimensions of Community Dental Health Abstracts
This abstract is sourced from the Professional Corpus, and is representative a number of language features commonly associated with professional writing of research reports in Community Dental Health. With a partner, can you label the highlighted text according to the following categories?

Present tense verbs
Evaluative Adjectives
Numbers and numerical conversions
Nouns and nominalisations
Passive voice constructions

Objectives: To identify the determinants of dental care utilisation [nominalisation] among Greek adults, with a particular emphasis on socio-economic determinants [nominalisation]. Methods: Data were collected [passive]through a national survey on health and health care services utilisation [nominalisation] of a sample of 4,003 Greek adults [numbers] stratified by geographic region, age and gender. A purpose made questionnaire was used [passive] during face-to-face interviews. A 2-stage model was developed [passive] to assess the impact of independent variables on dental utilisation likelihood and frequency [nominalisation]. Results: 39.6% (1,562) of Greek adults [numbers] reported having visited a dentist within the last year. Among dental attenders, 32.6% [numbers] reported prevention [nominalisation] as the reason for visit. Statistically significant [evaluative adjectives] differences in dental care utilisation [nominalisation] were observed in relation to demographic, socioeconomic and lifestyle factors. Logistic regression analysis showed that gender, age, income, education, place of residence, private insurance coverage and self-rated oral health are important [evaluative adjectives] determinants of dental services utilisation. Mean number of dental visits within previous year was 1.6 [numbers]. Results from Poisson regression analysis indicate [present tense] that lower income level correlates [present tense] to lower number of dental visits, while having visited for treatment (rather than for prevention) correlates [present tense] to higher number of dental visits. Conclusions: Greek adults do not exhibit [present tense] satisfactory [evaluative adjectives] dental visiting behaviour. Extent of care sought is [present tense] associated with need for treatment rather than preventive reasons. The findings confirm [present tense] the existence of socioeconomic inequalities in dental services utilisation among Greek adults.
Now, with the same partner, determine why professional writers might use these language features by matching the features to their function:

Language feature	Function
Nouns and Nominalisations	To be Authoritative and to convey stance [evaluative adjectives]
Evaluative adjectives	To condense information [nouns]
Passive constructions	To emphasise what was done, rather than who it was done to [passives]
Present tense verbs	To be impersonal and objective [numbers]
Numbers and numerical conversions	To be informative, stating findings as facts [present tense]

Figure 5.19 Corpus task 5-1

Corpus task 5–2 (see Figure 5.20) is inspired by the analysis of case reports in Chapter 4, and is related to the finding that these reports contain frequent reference to the expression of causality (the semantic field *A2.2 cause & effect / connection* was considered specific to case report writing). Students are directed to consult the professional corpus to explore the use of the causal expressions 'due to' and 'caused by', before consulting concordances to complete the next set of questions involving 'lead to', 'results in', 'based on', 'because of' and 'related to', each of which appeared frequently in the case report corpus.

Corpus task

Corpus task 5–2: Explaining the causes

These expressions are sourced from a corpus of dentistry Case Reports, although they are also frequently found in CHP writing:

Due to	*Results in*	*Caused by*	*Because of*
Based on	*Related to*	*Lead to*	*Hence*

Using the professional corpus, write 2 potential causes for dental issues that appear in the concordances for the following expressions:

1. … due to ____________________
2. … due to ____________________
3. … caused by ____________________
4. … caused by ____________________

Complete the following sentences by consulting concordances from the professional corpus

1. Oral prophylaxis *leads* to ______________
2. Tooth wear *results* in ______________
3. The analysis was *based* on ______________
4. Systemic complications that might arise *because of* ______________
5. Age and SES were also *related* to ______________

Figure 5.20 Corpus task 5-2

Corpus task 6 displayed in Figure 5.21 is sourced from the analyses of hedging and boosting devices performed on the learner and professional corpora in Chapter 3, and focus on the discussion and conclusion sections of the research report.

Question 1 in corpus task 6 uses hedging devices that were considered as specific to professional writing in the analysis in Chapter 3, including 'indicate', 'estimate', 'assume' and 'suggest', as well as the modals 'could' and 'may'. Students are guided to use the *frequency distribution* function, and the data will suggest in each case that these hedging devices are more likely to appear in the discussion function than in other sections of the research reports (Figure 5.22). This will allow students to answer the second part of this question once the table is complete.

Corpus task

Corpus task 6: Making reasonable claims/Hedging

1. Here is a list of commonly used hedging devices in academic writing. Work as a pair. Use the '*frequency distribution*' function to find out whether these hedging devices are most commonly used in the discussion section or other sections. Add an 'x' to the table when you find out the answer.

Hedging	Discussion section	Other section
Indicate		
Estimate		
Assume		
Suggest		
Could		
May		

2. These hedging devices tend to be overused by novice writers when writing CHPs. Can you replace the words in **bold** with an alternative expression?
   a. *Only* **about** *a quarter of the subjects* mentioned poor oral hygiene as a cause of decay
   b. There was **quite** a big difference when comparing the dental visit patterns of the studied Filipino domestic helpers …
   c. The poor oral health status of the children *is* **probably** *a result of* the limited public dental health program
   d. But **maybe** *it should not come as a surprise* that young adults prefer improving their appearance to their health care even in the presence of a minor toothache!

Figure 5.21 Corpus task 6

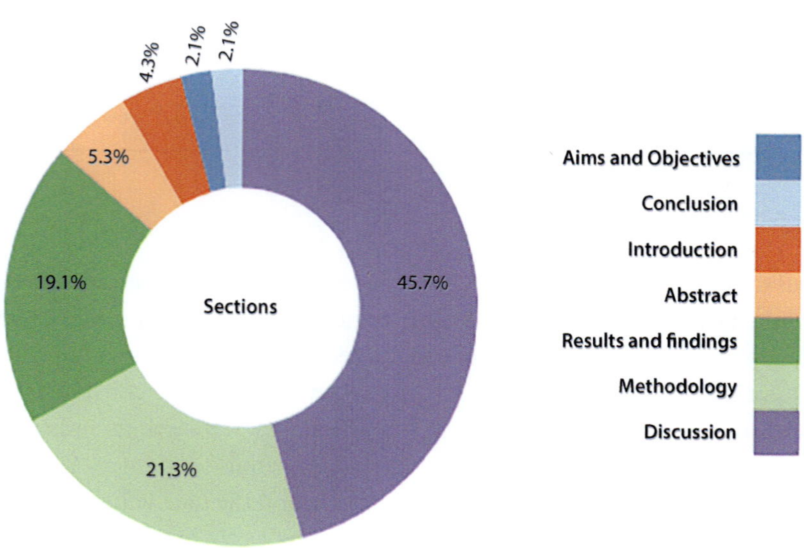

Figure 5.22 Frequency Distribution results for the hedging device 'indicate' in the learner corpus

Question 2 does not involve the direct use of the corpus, but involves four hedging devices that were found to be overused by novice writers in Chapter 3, including 'about', 'quite', 'probably' and 'maybe'. Students are instructed to replace these overused terms with synonyms.

Corpus task 7 (Figure 5.23) involves the use of boosting devices. The first question involves students using the corpus to learn how certain boosters tend to collocate with certain reporting verbs (and not with others). The second question involves a list of boosting devices taken from Hyland (2005), and which include

Corpus task

Corpus task 7: Using strengthening devices
Using the Learner Corpus, select the 'discussion' and 'conclusion' sections when answering the questions below:

1. **Which verbs usually collocate with these expressions? (enter the verb, then click collocation, noting the verbs to the right of the expression)**
   a. Strongly _
   b. Clearly __
   c. Definitely _
2. **Here is a list of words that can be used to strengthen claims. In pairs, use the professional corpus to work out whether these expressions are commonly used by counting the number of concordance results they generate, and by looking at their frequency information in the corpus. If you get time, compare the results in the professional corpus with the learner corpus.**

Actually	Always
Beyond doubt	Certain(ly)
Clear(ly)	Conclusive(ly)
Decidedly	Definite(ly)
Demonstrate	Doubtless(ly)
Establish	Evident(ly)
Find/Found	**In fact**
Indeed	**Know**
Indisputable(y)	Must
Never	No doubt
Obvious(ly)	Prove
Show	**Think**
Thought	Undeniably

3. **Based on your investigation of these boosting devices, which ones do you think you should use when making strong claims in the discussion and conclusion sections of your CHP reports?**

Figure 5.23 Corpus task 7

each of the 'overused' boosters by novice CHP writers in Chapter 3 (shown in **Bold**) as well as those boosters which were determined to be frequently used in professional writing (shown in *italics*, although neither the bold nor italics featured in the real task).

By querying the number of concordances generated from the data, as well as referring to the frequency information, students can then make data-informed decisions as to which boosting devices they can use when making claims, as they are directed to consider in Question 3. For example, only 21 hits are generated in the professional corpus data for 'think', compared with 127 hits in the learner corpus. When monitoring students, the ESAP tutor should comment as to why this difference in frequencies across the two corpora is important when considering the relative over/underuse of expressions between novice and professional writing.

5.6.1 Supplementary Moodle tasks

All students were also required to complete four supplementary tasks outside of class using the Moodle LMS. Three of these tasks used data derived from the analyses in Chapters 2 to 4. These focused on the functions of citation and effective use of citation verbs, choosing the appropriate tense for the method, results, and discussion sections, and additional activities on the use of hedging and boosting devices.

The activity on recognising different citation forms (Figure 5.24) was created as a result of the analysis conducted in Chapter 3 using the *Ubiqu+Ity* platform, which found the learner texts contained more frequent use of integral citations referring directly to the author of the claim in subject position, while in the professional texts, authors tended to use non-integral citations in order to avoid specific mention of the author, focusing instead of the claim. Aluthman (2017) found students exposed to DDL were able to reduce the amount of integral citations made while increasing their use of non-integral citations. While we did not develop activities on citation practices that required students to consult the corpus themselves or get them to use preferred citation patterns, the questions we designed involved students identifying different citation patterns using authentic examples derived from our corpus data.

The use of present tense forms in professional writing to present findings as facts was a feature of the MDA analysis in Chapter 3, as well as the finding in Chapter 2 that dentistry research reports often use present tense forms to describe methodological procedures that took place in the past, eschewing a narrative retelling of events for a more instructional tone. More examples of present tense verb use in professional writing were added to this supplementary activity, with students selecting the correct form of the verb from a drop-down menu (Figure 5.25)

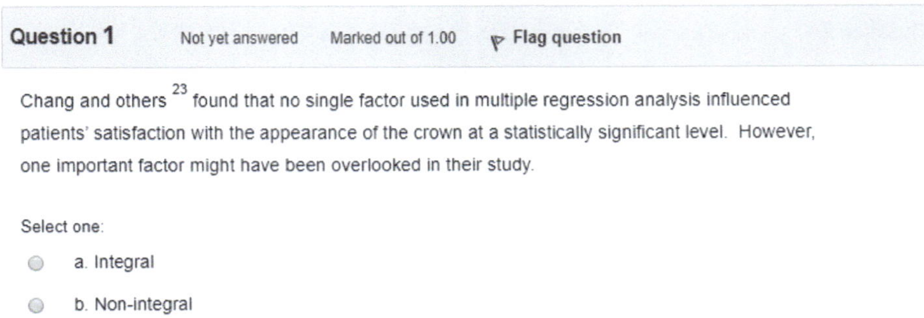

Figure 5.24 Supplemental activity on integral vs. non-integral citations

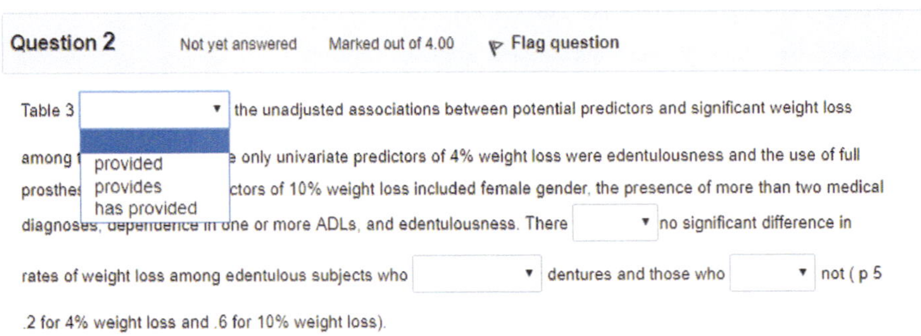

Figure 5.25 Supplemental activity on present tense verbs in professional writing

The supplemental task on hedging and boosting complements the other in-class corpus-based activities that address this function by exposing students to concordances from the professional corpus. Figure 5.26 describes how students were asked to explore adverb collocates of the booster 'significant' by reading the concordances, with suggested answers including 'clinically' and 'statistically'.

Question 2 Not yet answered Marked out of 2.00 Flag question

Identify and put down the **adverbs** that collocate with **"significant"** in the box provided below.

1. It remains uncertain despite **significant** advancement in medicine in
2. the increase in response was **significant** after patients watched the video
3. is considered to be clinically **significant.** All the participants in this
4. taken by people; it contributed **significant** amount to overall impression and
5. programme. Despite this, no **significant** change in the overall mean
6. the examination, there is no **significant** change in number of people
7. 13% in score 2 and again no **significant** changes were noted in the score 0.
8. non-invasive procedures. No **significant** correlation was found between the
9. In our study, we found that **significant** decrease in anxiety experiences
10. -square test), but a statistically **significant** difference between the test group

Answer:

Figure 5.26 Exploring 'significant' with concordances from the learner corpus

5.6.2 Additional activities

As some of the analyses in Chapters 2 to 4 were completed *after* the 2017–2018 cohort had begun, we later added two additional supplemental activities into the curriculum mid-way. Given the importance of the passive voice construction as a feature of disciplinary writing in Chapters 2 and 3, we developed the following two-part activity that first asked students to rewrite passages written in active voice in the passive voice, with examples taken from the professional corpus. Students then needed to search either the Professional or Learner Corpus using the query syntax "was *_v", followed by the *collocation* function, and write down five example sentences using any of the verbs derived from the output (Figure 5.27).

Corpus task

The passive voice in dentistry writing

A. **Rewrite the following sentences from the Professional Dentistry Corpus into passive voice:**
   1. We **administered** the questionnaire between May and July 2008, before DGA and face-to-face by one of the authors (AK), who recorded participant responses.
      [suggested answer] ***The questionnaire was administered*** *between May and July 2008, before DGA and face-to-face by one of the authors (AK), who recorded participant responses.*
   2. We **adopted** the level of $p < 0.05$ for statistical significance.
      [suggested answer] *The level of* $p < 0.05$ ***was adopted*** *for statistical significance.*
   3. The population assessed in the present study did not show a high score of enamel defects (Cypriano et al., 2003); however, there is no guarantee that enamel defects **affected** the occlusal surface or that all of them were stain-free.
      [suggested answer] *The population assessed in the present study did not show a high score of enamel defects (Cypriano et al., 2003); however, there is no guarantee that* ***any occlusal surface was affected*** *or that all of them were stain-free.*

B. **Search either the Professional or Learner Corpus using the term "was *_v", and use the 'collocation' function. Write down five sentences using any of the verbs you see in the results**
   [potential verbs] *Found; Conducted; Recorded; Performed; Assessed*

Figure 5.27 Supplemental corpus task 1

The second supplemental task was drawn from the sentiment and semantic analyses conducted in Chapter 4, aiming to raise student awareness of the general and disciplinary senses of dental terminology. It would have been preferable to get students to consult the professional Dental Public Health corpus for this activity, but expressions such as 'immature' and 'aspiration' had no hits in that corpus, and tended to maintain their general rather than disciplinary sense in the learner corpus data. As students did not have access to the case report corpus data used in Chapter 4, we instead hand-picked concordance lines from that data (using *AntConc*) that would clearly exemplify the stark difference between the disciplinary sense of these expressions and their general sense (Figure 5.28)

Corpus task

General and disciplinary senses of a word

A. Match the meanings of the words in left column to their meaning on the right

1. Immature	**a. Something you hope and dream for** [4]
2. Correct	**b. Another term for a test** [3]
3. Examination	**c. When you get the right answer** [2]
4. Aspiration	**d. Giving a speech in public** [5]
5. Presentation	**e. When someone is acting childish** [1]

F. The following concordance lines are taken from a corpus of Dentistry Case Reports. Can you add the words 1–5 above into the gaps? Add the number to the gap.

1. …borders of indication towards cariously exposed _[1]_ permanent teeth with reversible pulpitis
2. Osteopetrotic conditions vary greatly in their _[5]_ and severity, ranging from neonatal onset …
3. A submandibular fine-needle _[4]_ was performed confirming the diagnosis of "metastatic carcinoma."
4. Both clinical and radiographic _[3]_ confirmed the absence of permanent mandibular central incisors
5. Different techniques have been used to _[2]_ anterior and posterior crossbites …

G. Based on your answers to B above, what is the disciplinary meaning of these expressions?

1. Immature	**a. A procedure to straighten or repair** [2]
2. Correct	**b. A description of something (e.g. teeth) that is not fully grown** [1]
3. Examination	**c. The physical appearance of a disease or physical property of the patient** [5]
4. Aspiration	**d. Removal by suction of fluid and cells through a needle** [4]
5. Presentation	**e. An inspection of the teeth and surrounding soft tissues of the oral cavity** [3]

F. With a partner, discuss any other words you might know that have both a general meaning, and a special meaning in dentistry.

Figure 5.28 Supplemental corpus task 2

5.7 Chapter summary

This chapter has introduced how corpora have now become an essential component of 'writing-to-learn' in the context of ESAP. Despite the failure of the initial 'concordance only' run of the earlier ED materials, we believe that doubling-down on the corpus approach has now provided the necessary and sufficient conditions for students to experience the 'multiple affordances' of data-driven learning (Leńko-Szymańska & Boulton, 2015). The innovations in materials and technology described here have provided ED dentistry students with the tools and guidance needed to make crucial autonomous decisions about language as they engage with multiple data sources, following an active, constructivist approach to disciplinary composition, language and content learning. These pedagogical innovations now closely align with the Problem-Based Learning design element of the new dental curriculum, in which dentistry students are trained to take autonomous steps to tackle a problem, and to achieve their goals through sustained inquiry. In our case, students are resolving *language* problems, as realised through the PBL-like design of our DDL tasks, while at the same time achieving the overarching goal of understanding disciplinary discourses as part of 'writing to learn'. By carefully integrating bottom-up DDL activities with top-down structural and genre-focused tasks, we hope to have ensured a learner-centred focus-on-form (Bernardini, 2001; Fuentes, 2017) while avoiding Ädel's "most serious challenge" for DDL, that of a focus only on surface forms (2010: p. 52). We also feel our approach towards the design of DDL materials can be tailored to DDL-enhanced teaching of writing for other disciplines and genres, as long as you have a representative corpus and software that easily facilitates concordance, collocation and frequency information for queries, and we have already demonstrated this in other research (Crosthwaite, Wong & Cheung, 2019) and plan to work along similar lines for work involving pre-tertiary learners of English in the near future. Luckily, one does not require a purpose-built online corpus environment such as the one described in this chapter to achieve this – we have previously successfully designed similar activities on seasonal DDL courses using freely available software such as *AntConc, SketchEngine for Language Learning (SKELL),* or *SketchEngine* (the open version which includes BAWE) (see Crosthwaite, 2017, 2018 for descriptions of these previous activities). While good corpus tools certainly make the job easier, the best foundation for successful DDL is a good corpus, carefully designed tasks that allow students to both freely explore as well as constrain their corpus engagement (so as to avoid "drowning in data", Ädel., 2010: p. 45), and (perhaps most importantly) meaningful integration into the writing curriculum rather than being left at the periphery.

Were we eventually successful in our aims? This remains to be seen at the close of this chapter. Data on whether and to what extent our materials facilitated successful disciplinary DDL for dentistry writing are now reported in the next chapter.

CHAPTER 6

Putting it into (dental) practice

User engagement with dentistry corpora and DDL

6.1 Introduction

In Chapter 5, we reported on the construction and integration of our purpose-built online corpus platform into the ESAP ED course, and described a suite of in-class and out-of-class activities using this platform for the purposes of *Data-Driven Learning* (DDL, Johns, 1991). While the majority of DDL studies focus on student/ teacher perceptions of DDL or experimental work looking for improvements in accuracy or lexical knowledge, very little is currently known about students' corpus query habits during DDL for disciplinary writing purposes (Hafner & Candlin, 2007). This data is very important to disciplinary DDL studies in that "what students report to be doing or what we assume they are doing when we observe them might be quite distant from what they are actually doing" (Pérez-Paredes, Sánchez-Tornel, Alcaraz Calero, & Jiménez, 2011, p. 235).

Documenting students' corpus queries has typically been done manually (e.g. Chambers & O'Sullivan, 2004; Frankenberg-Garcıa, 2005), or through the collection of computer logs (e.g. Gaskell & Cobb, 2004; Hafner & Candlin, 2007; Yoon, 2008; Pérez-Paredes, Sánchez-Tornel, Alcaraz Calero, and Jiménez, 2011). Taking a manual approach, Chambers and O'Sullivan's (2004) study tracked corpus-assisted revisions made to the academic writing of eight advanced learners of French, asking students to document their corpus queries and revisions made to their work, while the Portuguese-English translation students involved in Frankenberg-Garcia's (2005) study were required to manually log the resources used to resolve translation issues including a selection of online concordance software. Taking a more automated approach, Gaskell and Cobb (2004) introduced a purpose-built platform to track students' error correction attempts, logging the number of corpus queries and IP addresses of users, although data regarding the syntax of the queries made or individual corpus usage habits was not collected. Later studies, particularly Hafner and Candlin (2007), Yoon (2008) and Pérez-Paredes et al. (2011) have been more successful in detailing actual corpus usage statistics and query syntax. Hafner and Candlin's study featuring students within the law discipline created a platform to track students' user IDs, date and time of access, users' search queries and the data on the corpora queried, albeit documenting only 248 queries over two years. Yoon (2008) also documented students' corpus use through the collection of query logs as well as data on time of usage from 10 corpus users in a qualitative study. Pérez-Paredes et al. (2011) collected data on individual corpus use, including the number of corpus activities completed, number of corpus queries produced, and data on the query syntax involved. However, there is still a great need for further detailed data on disciplinary writing students' corpus usage and query habits for DDL. This need is addressed here in Chapter 6, which focuses on categorising our dentistry ED students' cohort and idiosyncratic corpus engagement as they completed both the activities outlined in Chapter 5 and their CHP assignments.

6.2 Students' previous language reference habits

In order to be able to characterise students' corpus query behaviours during DDL, it is necessary to explore the different language reference resources that these students typically used prior to engagement with corpora, and whether they have in fact been exposed to corpora previously. Here, we present the results of a questionnaire first featured in Quinn (2014) that captures the language referencing habits of language learners prior to taking on DDL activities. Unfortunately, this data is taken from the 2016/2017 cohort, not the 2017/2018 cohort featured in the rest of the chapter. However, we seek to assure the reader that there will likely be very little difference in the responses given between these two cohorts in terms of the typical reference habits of Hong Kong university students, with similar results for HK postgraduate students already collected using the same questionnaire in Crosthwaite (2017). The questionnaire is divided into sections on *computer usage* and *writing reference tools*. There were 47 respondents in total for the 2016/2017 cohort.

Regarding computer usage, students were asked whether they liked to use computers, to which they responded positively (Yes=39, Sometimes=7, No=1). All 47 students reported that they use the internet at home, and all 47 reported that they are online almost every day, either through a PC or a smartphone. 28 respondents use a computer for school work almost every day, with 17 doing so three to four times a week, and with two students using a computer for school work just once a week. 43 respondents use a computer for personal purposes almost every day, with four respondents doing so three to four times a week. Students were then asked what percentage of their online activity was conducted in English, with 23 respondents claiming this was over 80%, nine respondents claiming between 60-80%, ten respondents claiming that about half of their online activity was conducted in English, and five respondents reporting percentages between 10–30%. To summarise, the student cohort are regular, typically online computer users who use this technology for both school work and personal use, and who primarily do so in English. Table 6.1 outlines students' responses to the second part of the questionnaire, focusing on writing reference tools.

Table 6.1 Student's pre-DDL use of writing reference tools

Question	Never	Rarely	Occasionally	Sometimes	Frequently	Usually
1. If you are unsure about vocabulary or grammar, how often do you use major Internet search engines (e.g. Google or Yahoo)?	0(0%)	3(6.4%)	7(14.9%)	5(10.6%)	16(34.0%)	16(34.0%)
2. How often do you use online translation sites to help you write in English?	9(19.1%)	16(34.0%)	9(19.1%)	9(19.1%)	3(6.4%)	1(2.1%)
3. When writing in English, how often do you use a portable electronic dictionary?	24(51.1%)	10(21.3%)	5(10.6%)	4(8.5%)	1(2.1%)	3(6.4%)
4. How often do you use online dictionaries?	0(0%)	7(14.9%)	8(17.0%)	13(27.7%)	15(31.9%)	4(8.5%)
5. How often do you use English-English monolingual dictionaries?	0(0%)	8(17.0%)	10(21.3%)	12(25.5%)	13(27.7%)	4(8.5%)
6. How often do you access smartphone apps for English referencing purposes?	12(25.5%)	14(29.8%)	6(12.8%)	3(6.4%)	9(19.1%)	3(6.4%)
7. How often do you use Microsoft Word's spellchecker or grammar checker?	4(8.5%)	3(6.4%)	9(19.1%)	10(21.3%)	14(29.8%)	7(14.9%)
8. How often do you use a thesaurus to help you with English vocabulary? (online or paper)	8(17.0%)	11(23.4%)	9(19.1%)	16(34.0%)	3(6.4%)	0(0%)
9. When you are unsure about grammar, do you use a grammar book / online grammar reference?	12(25.5%)	13(27.7%)	11(23.4%)	8(17.0%)	2(4.3%)	1(2.1%)
10. How often do you use an English language corpus to check vocabulary or grammar?	28(59.6%)	10(21.3%)	3(6.4%)	6(12.8%)	0(0%)	0(0%)
12. How often do you reference words or grammar points while you are writing?	12(25.5%)	14(29.8%)	9(19.1%)	8(17.0%)	3(6.4%)	1(2.1%)
13. When you are unsure about some language point, how often do you guess instead of confirming your grammar or vocabulary choice with a reference resource?	2(4.3%)	13(27.7%)	10(21.3%)	15(31.9%)	6(12.8%)	1(2.1%)

Regarding question 1, 26 students reported that they used an English-language search engine exclusively, four students reported using a non-English search engine exclusively, and 18 students reported using both English and non-English search engines. As for question 2, each student mentioned that Google Translate was the preferred software if they were to use translation websites. Regarding question 4, the most popular online dictionary used was Dictionary.com (16 students), followed by Google (8 students), followed by a range of other resources that were used by just one student each, including Iciba, Oalize, Merriam Webster, Medline, Naver, and the Cambridge online dictionary. Some of these appear to be mobile apps, which also feature in students' responses to question 6. A number of students said they used MS Word or Google in response to question 9 about grammar resources, with only one student saying they currently used *Grammarly*®. Question 11 (not shown in the table) asks students "Aside from the reference resources mentioned above, what other resources have you used to help you write in English?". Responses here were limited, but included 'ask someone who knows', 'native friends', and 'read samples/exemplars or similar articles'.

To summarise, the majority of students appear to use Google or other online English-to-English dictionaries as their go-to language reference resource. They do not generally refer to grammar resources, and about half of the cohort tend to 'guess' when faced with a language problem. Crucially, the response to question 10, relating to corpus use, is overwhelmingly negative, with 77.9% of respondents claiming they never or rarely used a corpus, although we are encouraged that 12.8% of respondents claimed they sometimes did use a corpus. When asked in a sub-question to question 10 whether students had 'ever heard of a corpus', eight respondents replied that they had, while 36 students replied that they had never heard of a corpus. The results from this questionnaire are very much in line with those already reported for Hong Kong postgraduate students in Crosthwaite (2017), and while these are the results from the 2016/2017 cohort, it is very unlikely that these results will have changed significantly. We do note, anecdotally at least, a sharp observed increase in the number of students turning to the error auto-correction tool *Grammarly*® at the time of writing this volume.

6.3 Learner behaviour tracking parameters and analysis

The corpus platform tracked learners' corpus use according to the following parameters: (1) User ID; (2) time, date and duration of user log-in to the platform; (3) individual corpus query syntax; (4) any filters applied to corpus query results (i.e. searches by thesis section), and; (5) corpus function used (i.e. concordance, frequency breakdown, etc.). The platform produced some of this data in a visual format (e.g. number of users, queries, query terms by frequency, while all five tracking parameters were output as .csv files which were analysed and summarised as seen in the results section by a bilingual speaker of English and Cantonese working as a research assistant on the project. As with Yoon (2008) and Pérez-Paredes et al. (2011), these parameters are considered 'precise' for corpus consultation as they allow for individual users' corpus use to be tracked instead of tracking by group. This data was intended to help the research team better understand which information learners are focusing on when querying the corpus, learn how users navigate the corpus to solve their language problems, and to assist with improvements to course content, the interface and its functionality in future iterations of the course. We also ensured that all teachers' usage histories and corpus queries were not included in the final results.

6.4 Total user engagement

The usage statistics across both professional and learner corpora are shown in Figure 6.1, taken directly from the learner analytics homepage. These span from the beginning of January 2018, when the second version of the corpus platform was released to the cohort, to the end of June 2018. The course ended at the end of April 2018, leaving two months post-course data collection in order to determine whether use of the corpus was maintained beyond completion of the course.

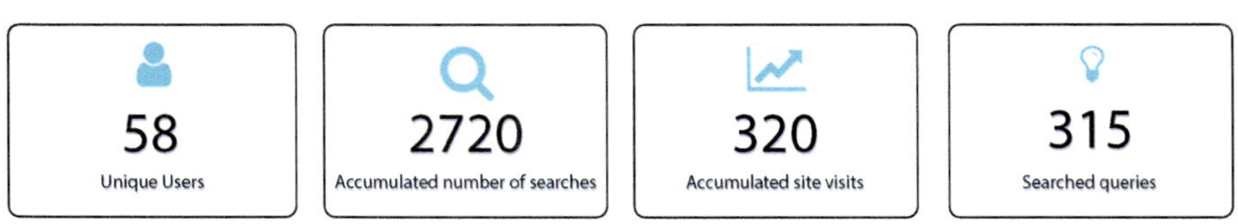

Figure 6.1 Usage statistics across both professional and learner corpora

Eight staff members were counted among the unique users in this figure, leaving 50 student users. One interesting point to note from these results is that the number of 'searched queries' (i.e. 'unique queries' = 315) is about one-eighth that of the accumulated number of searches (2,720), suggesting that the 50 student users of the corpus platform were often repeating a number of queries using the same query syntax. It is likely that a significant proportion of these 315 unique queries are presumably queries that were built-in to the corpus task materials – a finding we shall return to later. However, the number of unique queries is still much higher than those found within the course materials, meaning that students were, on the whole, often producing corpus queries that were of their own making.

The distribution of queries across learner and professional corpora (Table 6.2) is pre-determined, in part, in that the corpus tasks presented in the materials more frequently required the learner corpus to be queried as compared with the professional corpus. However, the proportion of unique to accumulated searches in the professional corpus is much higher (20.6%) than that of the learner corpus (11.9%), meaning that when the learners did consult the professional corpus, they were more likely to generate queries that were not already included in the corpus task materials. Students can be said, therefore, to be more freely experimenting with the data available in the professional corpus, when given the opportunity.

Table 6.2 Queries by corpus

Corpus	Unique searches	Accumulated searches
Professional corpus (CODRA)	118	571
Learner corpus (HKUCHP)	257	2,149

6.5 Queries by section (Learner corpus)

Table 6.3 describes the distribution of searches by section (e.g. literature review, methodology, etc.) across the learner corpus. The option to search by section was not built in to the professional corpus during the data collection period, therefore we are only concerned with the learner corpus in this section.

When searching by section, corpus users most frequently queried terms within the methodology, introduction, and aims and objectives sections. Corpus tasks 1 and 3 (Chapter 5) ask students to search specifically within the introduction and aims and objectives sections, while corpus task 2 asks students to select 'all' sections (using the 'default', unchecked setting). Corpus tasks 6 and 7 ask students to query the discussion and conclusion sections, leaving only corpus task 4 specifically requiring students to query the methodology section. The finding that almost 36% of student queries were carried out within the methodology section of the learner corpus is striking given that there was only one activity with eight target items to be queried in the methodology section in the course materials (corpus task 4). This is therefore highly suggestive that students were specifically interested in the language features of the methodology section (as compared with other sections of the research articles) when conducting their own corpus queries outside of the course tasks. From a course developer's perspective, such findings suggest a need to revise corpus task 4 by extending the list of target verbs, or adding extra corpus tasks focusing specifically on other frequent language features within the methodology section.

Table 6.3 Queries by section in the learner corpus

Section	Number of searches	Proportion
Methodology only	772	35.92%
Default	664	30.90%
Introduction + Aims & objectives*	224	10.42%
Abstract + Introduction + Aims & objectives + Literature review + Methodology + Results & findings + Discussion + Conclusion	129	6.00%
Introduction + literature review	123	5.72%
Introduction only	94	4.37%
Introduction + Aims & objectives + Literature review	45	2.09%
Abstract + Introduction + Aims & objectives + Literature review + Methodology + Results & findings	43	2.00%
Abstract only	23	1.07%
Discussion only	10	0.47%
Abstract + Introduction + Literature review	8	0.37%
Start**	4	0.19%
Aims & Objectives only	3	0.14%
Literature review only	2	0.09%
Results & findings + Discussion + Conclusion	2	0.09%
Abstract + Introduction + Aims & objectives	1	0.05%
Conclusion only	1	0.05%
Introduction + Discussion + Conclusion	1	0.05%

* '+' is used when multiple check boxes were selected for a corpus query.
** The 'Start' section appears to have been an error left over in a few of the corpus files.

6.6 Queries by function

Tables 6.4 and 6.5 describe the distribution of queries by function (e.g. collocation, frequency breakdown, etc.) across both professional and learner corpora, including statistics on *sort* functions. The corpus platform requires a 'basic search' to be conducted before the use of other functions, which results in the high frequency for this function in Tables 6.4 and 6.5, accounting for over 50% of searches in both corpora respectively. However, there was some minor variation across corpora in terms of the usage of the *collocation* and *frequency breakdown* functions, with *collocation* used more widely in queries involving the learner corpus, and *frequency breakdown* used more widely in the professional corpus. This variation is unlikely to be statistically significant however, with the proportional use largely similar across corpora. Learners very rarely utilised the *sort KWIC by left context (L1)* function in either corpus. This could potentially be due to the face that students were not specifically prompted to use this function in the course materials, although students were informed about this function by their course tutors after they had begun using the platform and could see the option to sort the concordances in the user interface. On the other hand, this finding is also strongly suggestive that sorting concordances to the left of the search query provides a very specific kind of output that students either (a) do not understand how to make use of, or (b) does not provide the kind of information that they are typically using the corpus to search for.

Table 6.4 Queries by function (Professional corpus)

Function	Number of searches	Proportion
Search	303	52.88%
Frequency breakdown	106	18.50%
Collocation	92	16.06%
Frequency distribution	72	12.57%
Sort KWIC by right context (including default setting)***	541	94.42%
Sort KWIC by left context (L1)	32	5.58%

*** We were not able to disambiguate specific 'Sort KWIC from Right context' searches from the default setting when collating this data, therefore only the data where students explicitly sorted the KWIC from the left hand context is of interest here.

Table 6.5 Queries by function (Learner corpus)

Function	Number of searches	Proportion
Search	1,093	50.86%
Collocation	419	19.50%
Frequency breakdown	393	18.29%
Frequency distribution	244	11.35%
Sort KWIC by right context (including default setting)	541	94.42%
Sort KWIC by left context (L1)	32	5.58%

6.7 Query logs: Learner corpus

Table 6.6 describes the most frequent corpus queries users conducted using the learner corpus. The list of terms in Table 6.6 has a cut-off of 5 matched queries from the corpus data. Query forms that were present as exemplars in the course materials are distinguished in Table 6.6 from those generated by the learners themselves, with the latter presented in bold. While it is apparent that the majority of the more frequent query forms involved exemplars from the course materials, a number of

Table 6.6 Most frequent query forms in the learner corpus

Term	Frequency of repeated queries	Term	Frequency of repeated queries
my	63	**presumably**	9
was *_v	58	**was_v given**	9
we	47	**was_v conducted**	9
investigate*	46	**insufficient**	8
our	38	**missing**	8
correct*	34	**lack**	8
use*	33	**was_v found**	8
studies have * that	32	**include_v**	8
few	31	**were_v**	7
investigate	29	**studies**	7
investigate *	28	correct	7
serve*	27	suggest	7
obtain*	27	conclusively	7
inmates	25	obtained	6
use *	25	**autistic**	6
studies have shown that	25	**was ***	6
little	23	Investigat*	6
augment*	22	I	6
undoubtedly	21	studies have * that	5
autism	20	**include***	5
inadequate	19	using	5
serve *	19	use	5
limited	18	**much**	5
no	18	few studies	5
correct *	15	**research_n**	5
obtain *	14	**inmate**	5
augment	14		
augment *	12		
the data	12		
was_v used	11		
* have shown that	10		
corrected	10		
more	10		

other query terms were not explicitly provided in the materials and were generated by the learners themselves. It is also apparent that there is some degree of experimentation regarding even the query terms that *were* provided in the materials. For example, the term 'correct' appears in corpus task 4, which asks students to use a wildcard search to derive morpho-syntactic variants of frequent verbs in their base form. However, both the base form (without a wildcard), and the past simple form ('corrected') also appear frequently in the search results, as students seemingly use these different query forms to confirm hypotheses generated by the output from the original supplied query ('correct*'). This is also the case for the term 'use', with additional frequent queries including 'used', 'using' and even 'was_v used', where learners were attempting to use the POS function to discover more about the term 'use' as part of a passive construction, but were doing so erroneously (the POS tag is redundant).. Searches for 'investigate' also included 'investigate *', 'investigate*' and 'investigat*', as students experiment with the different outputs that appear as the result of repositioning the wildcard in the search syntax. As the learners were not prompted in the materials to attempt this query type, the prevalence of these alternate queries in the data is again suggestive of learners experimenting with the corpus under their own initiative.

The term 'inmates' was searched for 25 times, with this term part of the CHP research focus for one of the 2017/2018 ED project groups focusing on the oral health status of inmates among local prisoners in HK. The terms 'autism' and 'autistic' also featured in the data, and come from a CHP report that evaluated the effect of behavioural interventions such as visual pedagogy and positive reinforcement towards improving the oral hygiene of autistic preschool children in Hong Kong. These frequent searches for a specific term in the learner corpus suggest that some students used the corpus as a kind of 'database' or dictionary that would allow them to determine whether these terms are relevant to their research and how they are used in context – a usage referred to in Section 6.10 of this chapter as well as in the student interviews in Chapter 7.

Given the data on the prevalence of the passive voice in dentistry writing as described in previous chapters, it is interesting to note the high frequency with which the query term 'was *_v' is found in the learner corpus query log history in the learner corpus. This query form was presented in the supplemental activity on this construction described in Chapter 5 and is the only time students were instructed about the use of POS tags in searches in the materials.[27]. The frequent use of this query and variant query forms such as 'was *', 'was_v used', 'was_ v given', 'was_v found' and 'was_v conducted' strongly suggests that students were particularly interested in searching for passive forms in the learner corpus. In fact, attempts such as 'was_v used' (without the wildcard) are actually syntax errors that do not actually require the use of the POS tag, but will give the desired output

27. Although students could have found out about the POS function by clicking a link to accompanying 'help' file on the platform, which explained its use. We have no data as to whether this actually happened or not.

regardless. POS tags are used appropriately for a few other queries however, such as specifying verb rather than noun forms in queries such as 'research_n', although their use is not particularly frequent.

The boosting device 'undoubtedly' also features in the query history, and was not included in the list of such devices in the relevant corpus task. The term is instead present in another (non-corpus) task which asks learners to categorise a list of adverbs and adjectives as either hedging or boosting devices, which suggests that the learners had consulted the corpus for this term without being explicitly prompted to do so. Similarly, the hedging device 'presumably' also appears in the search history despite not being included in the relevant corpus task, again featuring in the aforementioned non-corpus based task on hedges and boosters. Therefore, the evidence suggests that a number of corpus users were querying the corpus for information about terms outside of those provided in the corpus activities, using their own initiative to learn about the distribution and function of these terms in an autonomous manner.

A number of query terms related to quantity and quality also appear in the query log history. Queries related to quantity tended to involve low quantities, namely 'few', 'no', 'limited', 'lack', and 'missing', although the terms 'more', 'much' and 'include' also feature in the data. As for quality, the term 'lack' (as in 'lack of research') is common, as are the terms 'inadequate' and 'insufficient'. Some of these terms are listed in the materials when exemplifying how to create a 'research gap' as part of writing the literature review (i.e. pointing out the gap in other's contributions) and as part of writing the limitations section of the reports (i.e. pointing out the gap left by the author's own contributions). While the terms 'few' and 'little' are specifically mentioned in corpus task 3 on writing the literature review, there are no specific activities requesting the students use the other terms such as 'missing', 'limited', 'lack' 'inadequate' or 'insufficient'. Rather, these terms are found in certain reading sections in the materials, for example:

> Because the average number of natural teeth in this sample was relatively small (a mean of 17 among dentate subjects), inadequate power may have precluded our ability to detect the impact of tooth type and chewing-surface area.

The query log history therefore strongly indicates that students are choosing to query the corpus when encountering these terms in reading passages so as to gain more information about their function, usage and distribution, before (presumably) using these terms in their own academic writing. They are doing this without explicit prompting in autonomous fashion – a key tenet of the affordances of DDL for language learning.

6.8 Query logs: Professional corpus

Table 6.7 describes the most frequent queries users conducted using the professional corpus. The list of terms in Table 6.7 has a cut-off of 5 matched queries from the corpus data. As mentioned previously, there were fewer corpus tasks asking students to focus on the professional corpus than those within the learner corpus. An interesting finding from the query log history from the professional corpus is that query terms that were explicitly given in corpus tasks (e.g. 'studies have * that') for the learner corpus also find their way into the log history for the professional corpus as well. We also see query terms that were *not* explicitly provided in the corpus tasks and that feature frequently in the learner corpus also feature frequently in the professional data, including the quantity/quality terms such as 'none', 'lack', 'limited' and 'undoubtedly'. This suggests that certain learners were willing to explore the distribution and usage of these terms in the professional data, presumably to confirm any hypotheses generated about these terms from discoveries gained when using the learner corpus. As with the learner corpus, students were particularly interested in querying the professional corpus data for passive voice constructions, with 'was *' the most queried term in the corpus, and with 'was *_v' as the second most frequent query term. Finally, students appear to have consulted the professional corpus to explore whether the term 'data' is treated as a singular or plural expression, with both 'data was' and 'data were' featuring frequently in the search history. For the reader's information, 'data was' has a frequency of 40 per 1,000,000 words in this corpus, while 'data were' appears approximately 350 per 1,000,000 words. This finding would leave the students in little doubt as to the preferred form in academic writing.

Table 6.7 Most frequent query forms in the professional corpus

Term	Frequency of repeated queries	Term	Frequency of repeated queries
was *	64	data	9
was *_v	34	data was	7
few	21	limited	7
the data	15	research has *	7
inadequate	13	no	6
studies have * that	12	lack	6
inmates	11	none	6
little	9	data were	5
undoubtedly	9	little *	5

6.9 Corpus query habits: Top 10 users

Table 6.8 describes the usage history of the top 10 most frequent users of the professional corpus. The data here show that even among the top ten users of the professional corpus, there is a good deal of variation in their query habits. For example, there is variation in the frequency of the different corpus functions employed, with certain users (e.g. Rank 3) only using the *collocation* function alongside basic searches, while others (e.g. Rank 1, Rank 4) preferred to use the *frequency breakdown* function over the *collocation* function, and while others still (Rank 7, Rank 10) preferred the *frequency distribution* function. This is either an indication that certain users were looking for different information from the corpus, or that they better understood or had a preference for the format of the output they were receiving when using a given function. There is also variation in whether the users attempted to explicitly sort their KWIC contexts to the left and right after querying the corpus. As they were not prompted to sort their results in the materials, the finding that some users experimented with this function while others did not is again potentially suggestive of either (a) evidence of individual preferences with regards to the need for particular information from corpus results, or (b) certain users' willingness to experiment with the full range of corpus functions available to them.

There is also apparent variation in the query syntax employed between different users, with some users querying with whole words (e.g. 'data', Rank 5), or wildcards in place of words in set phrases (e.g. 'studies have * that', Ranks 4, 5, 7, 9 and 10), others employing wildcards at the end of words to look up information on the lemma (e.g. Rank 1), others using POS tags only (e.g. Rank 3), others interested in particular POSs (e.g. adverbs, Rank 8), others mostly looking for expressions under a specific function (e.g. the 'gap', Rank 9) and others employing both wildcards and POS tags in their corpus queries (Ranks 2, 4). The students ranked 2 and 4 in this list appear to be responsible for the 'was *_v' query syntax noted earlier, with both students perhaps working alongside each other to work out the best way to bring up a list of passive expressions. It is clear from this data that despite all students receiving the same input from the course materials, the top ten most frequent users were generally searching for different information from each other, and querying the corpus in different ways in a manner that was either (a) comfortable to them, or (b) provided them with the type of information they were explicitly interested in.

As with the professional corpus data, there appears to be substantial variation in the query habits of the top ten most frequent users of the learner corpus (Table 6.9). Certain users preferred the *collocation* function over others (e.g. Rank 3), with others preferring the *frequency breakdown* function (e.g. Ranks 1, 4), while

Table 6.8 Corpus query history of top ten users (professional corpus)

Rank by query freq.	Accumulated queries	Collocation	Freq. breakdown	Freq. distribution	Search	Sort	Remarks
1	76	7	19	7	43	All sorted by default.	Frequent search queries are 'research has *', 'collect*', 'augment*'. Only used wildcards but no POS tags.
2	67	8	9	8	42	Managed to sort by both L1 and R1.	Frequently searched 'was *_v'. Wildcards and POS tags were used separately.
3	47	17	0	0	30	All sorted by default.	Mostly searched 'was *_v' with a verb in past participle form. Only POS tags were used.
4	44	5	14	7	18	Managed to sort by both L1 and R1.	Mostly searched 'studies have * that' and 'few'. Wildcards and POS tags were used separately.
5	40	9	9	6	16	All sorted by default.	Frequently searched 'studies have * that' and 'data'. Only wildcards were used.
6	30	7	7	5	11	Managed to sort by both L1 and R1.	Frequently searched 'the data' 'indeed'. Only wildcards were used.
7	27	5	6	8	8	All sorted by default.	Frequently searched 'studies have * that', 'little'. Only wildcards were used.
8	24	5	4	2	13	All sorted by default.	Searched 'studies have * that' and other adverbs often. Only wildcards were used.
9	24	5	5	4	10	Managed to sort by both L1 and R1.	Searched items related to literature gap (e.g. '* have shown that', 'little'). Only wildcards were used.
10	23	1	8	8	6	All sorted by default.	Searches were mostly limited to 'studies have * that'. Only wildcards were used.

Table 6.9 Corpus query history of top ten users (learner corpus)

Rank by query freq.	Accumu-lated queries	Collo-cation	Freq. break-down	Freq. distri-bution	Search	Sort	Remarks
1	113	20	30	13	50	All sorted by default	Highly interested in methodology, introduction, aims and objectives. Used wildcards but no POS tags. Mostly searched for (possessive) pronouns.
2	106	28	6	10	62	Managed to sort by L1 and R1	Mostly interested in abstracts. Used wildcards and POS tags separately. Mostly searched 'disabled children' and 'autism'. Also often searched for personal names.
3	103	30	13	6	54	Mostly sorted by default, rarely with L1	Mostly interested in methodology. Used wildcards and POS tags separately. Highly interested in the copular verb 'was *_v'.
4	102	27	33	17	25	Mostly sorted by default,rarely with L1	Highly interested in methodology, introduction, aims and objectives. Mostly looked for 'investigate*' and other verbs 'collect*' 'obtain*' in methodology. Only used wildcards but no POS tags.
5	87	25	14	14	34	All sorted by default	Mostly interested in introduction, aims and objectives. Interested in environmental related terms, as well as formulaic patterns (e.g. 'studies have * that'). Wildcards and POS tags were used separately.
6	78	19	27	25	7	All sorted by default	Interested in all sections. Mostly searched 'studies have * that'. Only wildcards were used.
7	74	7	20	8	39	Managed to sort by L1 and R1	Interested in methodology section.Mostly searched 'investigate*' and passive verbs collocated with the copular 'was *_v'. Wildcards and POS tags were used separately.
8	72	11	12	7	42	All sorted by default	Mostly interested in methodology, with occasional searches in all sections. Mostly looked for passive verbs collocated with the copular using an erroneous string 'was_v'. Wildcards and POS tags were used separately.
9	69	12	7	11	39	Mostly sorted by default, rarely by L1	Mostly interested in methodology and introduction. Looked for collocates of 'studies'. Wildcards and POS tags were used separately.
10	66	8	16	3	39	Mostly sorted by default, rarely by L1	Mostly interested in methodology. Mostly looked for passive verbs collocated with the copular using an erroneous string 'was_v'. Wildcards and POS tags were used separately.

others still made heavy use of the *frequency distribution* function (e.g. Rank 6). Corpus users also varied in their use of the *sort* function, with some never using this function (Ranks 1, 5, 6 and 8), some occasionally sorting left (Ranks 3, 4, 9 and 10), and others comfortable sorting both left and right (Ranks 2 and 7). Querying by section is also a major source of variance, with some users interested in single sections only such as the methodology (Ranks 1, 3, 7 and 10) or the abstract (Rank 2), with others searching via multiple sections at the same time (Ranks 4 and 5) and with others using the default option to search across all sections of the research report (Rank 6).

There is even more significant variation in the corpus query syntax strings employed among these frequent users in the learner corpus than seen in the professional corpus data. Users varied in their usage of wildcards and POS tags, with some using only wildcards (Ranks 1, 4 and 6), or a combination of wildcards and POS tags (Ranks 2, 3, 5, 7, 8, 9 and 10). The actual terms queried also vary significantly across these top users. For example, the most frequent user of the learner corpus mostly searched for pronouns, which feature in corpus task 1, although they also frequently searched for possessive pronoun forms, which did not feature in the materials. The second-ranked user tended to search for specific terms including 'disabled children' and 'autism' as well as personal names, none of which feature in the corpus tasks presented in the materials. The user ranked 5 in the list also searched for specific terms related to the environment rather than dental terms, which we are unable to account for. A number of users (Ranks 3, 7, 8 and 10) most frequently searched for passive constructions, with a number of them continuing to search using the 'was *_v' string, the string 'was *' or on occasion the erroneous string 'was_v'. The use of the latter string is strong evidence that learners within a DDL situation may actually share query strings with each other in classroom situations, with potentially negative consequences if the string that is shared is in fact erroneous or redundant. This is a finding that has so far not been reported in the DDL literature to date.

6.10 Corpus usage history: Activity logs

One useful function of the user analytics function built into the corpus platform is the ability to track individual platform usage by date and time. This allows us to generate an 'activity log' of the users' corpus usage habits as they log in and out of the corpus platform, which we can use to characterise their corpus usage style over time. We now present a detailed characterisation of the corpus usage history of the top four users of both professional and learner corpora (combined), as derived by triangulating their log-in information and their corpus query habits. We label each one according to a broad generalisation of their corpus usage habits across the duration of the data collection period.

6.10.1 Case 1: The 'abstract' thinker

15/01/2018: The user spent around half an hour experimenting with the learner corpus, starting with simple searches and gradually trying out new functions such as frequency distribution and collocation. The user began querying key terms including 'autism' 'autistic' and personal names, and the user began to signify the part-of-speech of query items (e.g. 'study_n'). Most search results were filtered by the section choice 'abstract'. At 07:41, the user briefly switched to the professional corpus for one search. At 15.50 in the afternoon, the user spent a minute blending the use of the three main query functions.

22/01/2018: The user's searching habits appeared to change when searching in the professional corpus – the user began by exploring collocations, frequency breakdown and frequency distribution functions before returning to simple searches. This time, wildcards were extensively used in substituting each possible word in the phrase 'studies have * that'. Concordance sorting remained R1 (default). However the user only spent ten minutes using the professional corpus here.

05/02/2018: The user spent about an hour on the learner corpus alone, focusing mostly again on the abstract. Simple searches, collocations and frequency breakdowns functions were used. This time, the most frequent search query was 'was *_v'.

19/02/2018 This was the final time the user logged into the learner corpus after not using it for a month. They spent around four minutes on searching for (and finding collocates of) the expressions 'conclusively' 'obvious' and 'appears to be', again mostly in the abstract section

This user began with the specific aim of filtering their queries within the abstract section of the learner corpus, even though they were not specifically guided to do so at any point while completing the corpus task materials. They continued to primarily search within the abstract section whenever they were querying the learner corpus on their subsequent visits, as they went through the various query terms outlined in the corpus tasks (e.g. 'studies have * that'). It is possible that the student was already working on the abstract section of their project when they were consulting the corpus, or were perhaps apprehensive about writing the abstract if they lacked experience in writing them, although we are unable to confirm these possibilities.

6.10.2 Case 2: The switcher

15/01/2018: The user alternated between the learner and the professional corpus. After spending two minutes conducting some simple searches in the professional corpus, the user spent another two minutes querying the learner corpus. The major search items were related to 'more' and 'few'. Then, the user alternated the corpus choice every three hits, jumping from professional to the learner and then back to the professional and learner and so on. Searches on this day were all basic search functions but the user learned the trick of narrowing down returned hits with the help of the section filter (i.e. introduction, abstract, aims and objective) in the learner corpus.

17/01/2018: The user just spent a minute, first on the learner corpus, and then on the professional corpus, using only basic searches for words beginning with 'nano'.

22/01/2018: The user spent 20 minutes solely on the learner corpus, mainly searching 'research has *' and going back and forth between simple search, collocation, frequency breakdown and frequency distribution. No specific section filtering or L1 sorting was used.

05/02/2018: Although the user spent just 36 minutes querying the corpus, 86 hits were recorded in a single visit. The user spent the first three minutes on the professional corpus with a strong focus on methodology, looking at simple concordance results and frequency breakdown information for 'augment*' and 'collect*'. The next four minutes were spent on the learner corpus instead, the user kept exploring the collocation, frequency breakdown and simple concordance lines using the same strings – 'augment*' and 'collect*'. For the next thirty minutes, the user returned to the professional corpus to search for the following strings– 'collect*' and variants of 'was *_v' (including 'was_v used' 'was_v given' 'was_v conducted').

12/02/2018: The user mostly conducted simple searches for 'the data*' in the learner corpus, with the last two minutes spent on 'the datum' in the professional corpus.

With the exception of the entry from the 22nd January, this student frequently switched between the learner and professional corpora when conducting their queries throughout the data collection period, again despite not being prompted to do so (in this manner at least) in the course materials. While it appears from the data that the student mainly went through the corpus tasks as instructed, rarely deviating from these except for querying terms beginning with 'nano', the data appears to suggest this learner felt it necessary to compare or confirm the findings generated from their queries in one corpus with those of the other corpus.

6.10.3 Case 3: The quitter

15/01/2018: The user spent the first 22 minutes looking up first person pronouns in the learner corpus. At first the user filtered results by introduction and objectives, but later on expanded the scope of search to cover more sections. Collocation and frequency distribution were briefly checked. In the next hour, the user went onto search and explore the three main functions in the professional corpus. Major queries included 'studies have * that', 'autism', 'oral health' and 'few'.

05/02/2018: This day the user spent an hour solely on learner corpus. The user first used wildcards to look for hits of verbs such as 'collect', 'choose', 'include', 'analyse' with wildcards, and then repeated the procedure with a POS tag '_v' instead. All searches and exploration of functions were limited to the methodology section.

12/02/2018: The user only spent 3 minutes on the search query 'the data', first in the learner corpus and then the professional corpus.

19/03/2018: It has been a month since the user's last use of both corpora. The user spent 8 minutes first on learner corpus, then professional corpus, and then back to the learner corpus. It is interesting that the user first conducted simple searches in the learner corpus, continued the basic search in the professional one, and finally explored the three other functions when s/he returned to the learner corpus. Most queries concerned hedges like 'likely' 'presumably' as well as boosters such as 'undoubtedly' 'conclusively' 'indeed'

This user began their exploration of the two corpora in earnest, conducting a great number of searches for terms both contained in the corpus tasks and of their own making, and spending two and a half-hours total across their first two visits. However, from the 12th February onwards, their corpus use ceased, and it was not until over a month later that they revisited the corpus to search for hedges and boosters, although these final searches were all conducted within a relatively shorter timeframe than seen in their initial efforts. Their final visit appears to be later than that of the others, which would have been at the stage where the students were drafting their CHP reports. Therefore, while their decision to drop the use of the corpus is disappointing, the finding that they later returned to use the corpus for a specific purpose is encouraging.

6.10.4 Case 4: The perfectionist

15/01/2018 The user spent the first 22 minutes looking up concordances of first-person pronouns in the professional corpus, with the introduction section checked.

22/01/2018 The user spent the first minute exploring the collocates and frequency distribution of 'studies have * that' in the professional corpus, and then spent another 6 minutes checking the frequency breakdown of 'studies have * that' in the learner corpus before looking up the frequency breakdown of 'few' in the same corpus.

28/01/2018 On this day, the user spent 2 hours mostly exploring the language patterns of 'study'. The sequence went from learner to professional and then back to learner corpus. The user tried sorting by L1 and R1 from time to time.

29/01/2018 The next day, the user briefly searched for collocates of 'research has' in the professional corpus.

05/02/2018 The user spent 43 minutes solely checking 'investigate', 'augment*', 'was *_v' in the methodology section of the professional corpus.

12/02/2018 A week later, the user briefly looked up the frequency distribution and breakdown of 'data' in the learner corpus.

This student had very clear goals about the particular terms they were querying during each visit, beginning with query terms found in the corpus tasks (e.g. first person pronouns, 'studies have * that'), but then conducting very specific searches mostly on single lexical items on later visits. The time spent and variety of searches involving these items is comprehensive, particularly for the entry listed on the 28th January where the learner spent 2 hours querying the term 'study' and using every function across both corpora to gain as much information as possible about this term.

6.11 Chapter summary

The findings of this chapter represent what is likely one of the most comprehensive analyses yet conducted on students' corpus queries and usage habits for DDL within an individual discipline. Similar to Hafner and Candlin (2007), we have found a high degree of individual variation in the uptake and query habits of the corpus users. We note that students varied in whether they accessed domain-specific knowledge, language-specific knowledge, or both. This data can also be used to guide future iterations of the corpus study materials so as to ensure the corpus and corpus activities meet the needs of all students in terms of the specific issues (domain, language) they may be having with their writing (Anthony, 2016). Individual variation was evidenced in particular by the users' activity logs, which allowed for a detailed, qualitative analysis of longitudinal development in corpus use. This data allowed us to experience users' successes and/or failures in using the corpus, as well as the modifications they made to their corpus query habits and usage over time.

It appears that DDL students often go beyond the provisions of their assigned DDL tasks to freely experiment with the data available. This was also found in Hafner and Candlin's (2007) study, where corpus consultation was an "integrated and self-directed part of the students' writing process, unconstrained by the imposition of specific data-driven learning tasks set by the teacher" (p. 316). We have also seen that some users regularly confirm and compare their findings from one corpus with that of another, and determined that the methodology section of the research report is a particular area of concern for our disciplinary students, with that section featuring heavily in the corpus usage statistics.

We may have provided the tool, materials and training, yet we have been surprised at the level of innovation shown by the student cohort as they went beyond the provisions of the course materials to generate queries and interpret corpus results under their own autonomy. We are particularly surprised at the short length of time required for training students to use the corpus platform successfully, particularly as students on previous small-scale DDL courses conducted by the research team (and using publically available corpus platforms) required extensive amounts of training before users could conduct basic wildcard or POS searches, not to mention collocation or frequency-based functions (Crosthwaite, 2017). This early success was also the case in our study using the current corpus platform for multidisciplinary post-graduate thesis writing (Crosthwaite, Wong & Cheung, 2019). We credit this success to the careful design and planning of the corpus tasks outlined in Chapter 5, which was made easier through the user-friendliness and highly visual nature of the corpus query platform. Complicated or unappealing corpus query tools are, in our opinion, one of the biggest hurdles for the successful uptake of DDL because they constrain the types of learning activities that can and cannot be performed in the classroom, and eventually require much more in the way of teacher-led guidance and training. Our results in this chapter show that if the corpus platform is intuitive enough, and the DDL tasks sequenced appropriately with clear instructions, then there is less need for teachers to devote precious in-class time to guided instruction and drills on corpus consultation.

The data we have uncovered in this chapter, in turn, provides the research team with an insight into the strengths and weaknesses of the platform that can be used in future iterations. For example, we can see that not all users engaged with the corpus frequently, with a number never actually using the platform at all, and with a large number of users dropping the corpus after a short period of time. The accumulated frequency of corpus queries among even the most frequent users ranged between 60 to 70 for the learner corpus and 90 to 100 in the professional corpus, which strikes us as rather low across an entire course, although the range of corpus queries conducted outside of the specifications from the course materials does suggest students are not just using the corpus to complete the set activities. Disappointingly, despite the positive results from the usage data provided in this chapter, one particularly telling statistic from the data is that there were almost no searches made once the course was completed in April 2018, within either the learner or professional corpora. Granted, the students will have completed their submission of the CHP capstone report towards the end of April, with no further written assessments imposed on them between May and June, our two month window for post-course data collection. The students would also have likely lost their access to the corpus platform shortly after June. However, the finding that no more than 10 searches were conducted during the immediate post-course data collection between April and June is worrying. This is potentially suggestive of a failure to maintain sustained involvement with the corpus as a reference resource, with students returning to their preferred translation websites once the course was complete. We return to this issue in Chapter 7.

One limitation of this chapter that must be mentioned here is that as the students had graduated shortly after completing their Community Dental Health projects, we were unable to contact the individual students featured in the top ten lists, or the four students featured in the activity logs, to ask them *why* they decided to use the two corpora in the manner that they did. We also did not interview the students *as* they made their queries, as the students were free to complete many of the activities out of class. Therefore, we can only make assumptions about students' true intentions behind their corpus use based on the search history data as they used the two corpora. Another limitation, as mentioned previously, was that the functionality to search by section in the professional corpus was not implemented in time for the 2017/2018 cohort to make use of it, although it will be interesting to compare the learner/professional usage statistics in this regard in future research. It might also be useful to look at the breakdown of corpus queries and usage per activity type so as to see expected search behaviour vs. triggered search behaviour, at least for the activities conducted in class. As the platform only records queries, IDs and filter analytics, matching queries to corpus activities would have to be done manually, which would be difficult given the data structure of the user analytics and the high number of corpus searches. This also made it impossible to generate usage durations for all users without taking an inordinate amount of time to checking each individual corpus query, the time it was made, the time between the next search, the time logged in, etc. for each user. We are therefore limited to the four qualitative descriptions of corpus usage outlined in this chapter in this regard. It might also be useful in the future to look at the breakdown of corpus queries and usage per activity type so as to see expected search behaviour vs. triggered search behaviour, although this was impossible in our case given the structure of the data as it is collected in real-time. Nonetheless, we are still confident that the findings of this study represent a detailed insight into students' disciplinary corpus use for DDL, while highlighting the affordances of such use for those looking to implement DDL into their own practice.

CHAPTER 7

Reflections on practice, and future directions

7.1 What did we do, and what did we learn?

In this volume we have created a range of corpora and used a variety of corpus tools in a bid to reveal the language features underlying the discursive practices of dentistry writing. Using the findings of these corpus-based investigations, we were then able to successfully generate a range of materials with the aim of teaching the 'language of dentistry' to future dentists. Despite not being subject experts in the dentistry discipline, our presentation of the findings contained in this volume means that we can no longer consider ourselves "reluctant dwellers in a strange and uncharted land" (Wu & Badger, 2009: p. 20) as we were at the outset in Chapter 1. What we found and (more importantly) what we learned are now the focus of this section.

Our investigation of the experimental research report genre across general medical and dentistry disciplines in Chapter 2 uncovered a trend of frequent passive voice constructions in both corpora, but in particular in writing for the dentistry discipline. The prevalence of these constructions constrains the selection of other linguistic features of the writing including verb tenses, pronouns, and participles. Significant variation in the use of narrative features, passive constructions, and perfect constructions was also found across different key journals publishing research reports within the dentistry discipline. We discovered that published writers of high-impact dentistry research writing tend to present the findings of others (and themselves) as facts, through the use of predictive modals, conditionals, and demonstrative pronouns, and tend to categorise patient types through the addition of explicit information following WH-pronouns. We have also derived teachable discipline-specific lists of words and phrases common to the research article genre that either featured directly in ESAP course materials, or at least are set to feature in future iterations of the course. While our focus was necessarily on dentistry, we feel the tools and approach taken in Chapter 2 can be applied to any discipline, as long as the researcher has access to good, representative corpus data. Such tools (e.g. the *MAT tagger*) also make the task much easier for those embarking on their initial forays into register analysis, regardless of the overall descriptive or pedagogical aims of such research.

Our corpus-based comparison of learner and professional research report writing in the field of Dental Public Health in Chapter 3 has provided a wealth of insights on novice disciplinary writing, which were in turn used to enhance ESAP provision for novice dentists also tasked with writing for this genre. Significant variation was found between novice and professional reports in terms of narrative features, language features associated with explicit persuasion, a tendency to make tentative claims, active voice constructions, and a focus on animate referents – with each of these more likely to be found in novice attempts at this form of research report writing than found in professional writing. The tendency for tentativeness is also exhibited in the frequency and wordings of hedging and boosting devices present in the novice texts, and the narrative, active nature of novice writing is also seen in the prevalence of self-mention exhibited by these student writers. We have also conducted automated analyses of rhetorical features in the learner data, noting that student writers frequently provide additional background information as to the physical setting of the research and the properties of their research participants, frequently liken their research to that of a journey, and have a preference for citing others' research by referring directly to the author. Based on these findings, we recommended that ESAP tutors need to provide explicit instruction on the discursive norms and rhetorical expectations of writing in the disciplines. This instruction can be greatly enhanced by providing students with the technology through which they can meaningfully compare their own written work with that of the norms of their target discipline.

Our volume has also provided novel, corpus-based *and* corpus-driven insights into the sentiment and semantic features of the dentistry case report genre in Chapter 4. Using software still largely untested in the field of ESAP research, we found a set of terms used to convey positive and negative emotions in general English but which are used in an alternative disciplinary sense in case reports. We have also realised that case reports tend to focus much more on patients than research reports do, with the implication that novice writers of this critical disciplinary genre need to be aware of this from the outset. We have also determined that lexis and phraseology related to the semantic domains of measurement, comparisons, expressions of time, and descriptions of substances and methods are all crucial elements of reporting on patients and procedures within authentic dentistry cases. This finding implies that specific instruction in these semantic domains, while presumably missing from current practice, can and should be part of the dental ESAP curriculum. We believe that the impartial, corpus-driven perspective to disciplinary lexis adopted in Chapter 4 can help shed new light on other disciplinary genres and registers that have already received extensive treatment in the applied linguistics literature, such as research articles or narratives. Such NLP-driven analyses are already a major focus of a whole branch of computational linguistics research into medical health text mining as described in Chapter 1. However, their application in academic writing research and pedagogy is still sorely lacking, despite very recent new research (Whiteside & Wharton, 2019) and the efforts of researchers in developing accessible tools for such research (e.g. Kyle & Crossley, 2015; Crossley, Kyle & McNamara, 2016). We therefore hope Chapter 4 is a step in the right direction for this approach, particularly for L2 learners who not only have to acquire disciplinary vocabulary but may have more trouble dealing with polysemous disciplinary and non-disciplinary senses of such vocabulary. In addition, distant reading approaches such as the semantic analysis reported in Chapter 4 stand to greatly assist with the discovery of a range of frequent functions that may be hiding in plain sight within previously well-researched disciplinary genres and registers.

Based on the knowledge gained from our corpus-based analyses of three key genres of dentistry disciplinary writing, we developed a purpose-built corpus query platform with a suite of accompanying pedagogical tasks that have created the opportunity for our novice dentists to engage – as we have done – with the language features of disciplinary writing. The corpus platform and activities outlined in Chapter 5 were designed to allow novice dental writers to focus on domain- and language-specific lexis and phraseology, while developing the digital literacy skills required to query disciplinary corpus data under their own autonomy. In a major improvement to the concordance-focused approach of previous iterations, students were guided to query, interpret and evaluate a variety of visual and statistical data, and then to draw on these multiple sources of information when making decisions about language in use. We have extended the problem-based learning approach of their disciplinary content provision to that of resolving problems with their academic writing, and this has been done without the need for lengthy, explicit training on corpus use by an 'expert' in corpus linguistics.

Finally, in Chapter 6, we were able to discover – likely for the first time in the literature at this level of detail – how disciplinary writing students for dentistry *actually* engage with data-driven learning. We found that DDL students often go beyond the provisions of their assigned DDL tasks and will, if given the opportunity, freely experiment with the data available. This freedom to experiment leads to significant variation in the adoption of particular corpus functions and the query syntax typically adopted by users, in that students varied in whether they accessed domain-specific knowledge or language-specific knowledge. We have seen that users regularly confirm and compare their findings from corpus to corpus and function to function. We have also outlined four distinct trends in the individual usage characteristics of students as revealed by their detailed activity logs, although we are aware there are likely other approaches to users' corpus usage that we have not detailed within this volume. This essential data, as well as other findings revealed in Chapters 2 to 4 that we were unable to incorporate in the ESAP study materials at the time of writing, is already being used to develop future versions of the corpus study materials. This work will ensure the provision of high quality, research-based, and data-driven activities that work to promote the necessary conditions for 'writing-to-learn' to become manifest in our ESAP provision.

7.2 Did it work?

> Provided that learners adopt the appropriate instruments and methodology to actually be able to perform language research, are the results worth the effort?
>
> (Gavioli, 2005, p. 29)

From the authors' point of view, our investigations and pedagogical innovations outlined in Chapters 2 to 6 have, for the most part, resulted in a positive answer to Gavioli's question posed above regarding corpora and ESAP pedagogy. Through this volume, we have been able to share our findings with the ESAP and corpus linguistics research communities regarding the language features present within key genres in dentistry writing and the affordances of DDL for ESAP provision. We also have a tried-and-tested ESAP course, now fully updated with the latest pedagogical innovations in data-driven learning and with further data-driven improvements to course content on the horizon. We have an intuitive, visually appealing and multi-functional purpose-built corpus platform that has already featured in other related research on postgraduate thesis writing courses (Crosthwaite, Cheung & Wong, 2019) and which will be modified for use in other corpus-related projects in the future, notably for projects on data-driven learning with younger primary and secondary-aged learners. We do hope to eventually make this platform open source, so as to share it with the wider research community. Given the above, we feel that the immediate goals of the volume have been met. However, for the provisions of this volume to truly be considered successful, we must consider the opinions of the other stakeholders involved, namely the students themselves, the other ESAP tutors who taught students on the course, and the disciplinary tutors from the Faculty of Dentistry. We now focus on each of these groups of stakeholders in turn.

7.2.1 Student evaluation of DDL

The student cohort completed two questionnaires administered centrally by the university with regards to the ED course (the *Standards of Excellence in Teaching and Learning* [SETL] and the *Course Quality Questionnaire* [CQQ]), and an additional questionnaire based on Yoon and Hirvela (2004) focusing specifically on their DDL experiences. Regarding the SETL scores for course effectiveness, these improved from a 55.8% satisfaction rate from the previous cohort, to as high as

70.8% for the most recent cohort as taught by the second author (who was the course coordinator of the ED programme), indicative of a major improvement in students' reported perceptions of the course. There was a 3.3% rise for the programme as a whole, with a response rate of 88.2%. Moreover, the SETL teacher effectiveness scores were at 83.9% for this cohort, a raise from the previous year of 3%. The results for the Course Quality Questionnaire (CQQ) were also encouraging, with a small increase in satisfaction under the criteria "Use appropriate language to present research findings based on relevant review of literature, research methods, data collection, and recommendations" from 67.2% to 68.2%. There was no change in the results for the criterion "Deploying strategies for research report writing and apply these when writing different sections of a report" (67% satisfied). There was, however, an increase in score for the criterion "The eLearning resources (e.g. Out-of-class Learning Modules on the Moodle site, Dentistry Corpus Search) have provided useful support for self-directed learning", which garnered only a 42.8% satisfaction rate in 2016/2017, but rose to 51.7% for the 2017/2018 cohort. The response rate to the CQQ was also 88.2%. While the CQQ scores are still low overall (as with the overall SETL course effectiveness scores), there were no apparent specific comments about the corpus tasks or platform at all, with student dissatisfaction instead focusing on issues related to course workload, and classes running for too long. As qualitative comments are optional for both the SETL and CQQ, students who actively leave qualitative comments on these questionnaires tend to leave negative comments, with only a few positive comments typically reserved for the teacher. We therefore tentatively take the students' silence regarding the corpus platform in the CQQ to be a positive sign, especially given the numerous negative comments levelled specifically at the corpus platform and activities following the first unsuccessful iteration of these into the ED course in the previous year.

Due to an administrative error, our version of Yoon and Hirvela's (2004) post-DDL questionnaire was sent out *after* students had graduated, meaning that only 2 students from the course returned the completed forms. With this in mind, we instead interviewed these students for their opinions on the corpus platform and activities, and asked them whether they perceived these to be useful for disciplinary writing. The students' overall impressions of the DDL component of the course was that it was 'very useful'. Student A felt that this component would work better in an entirely out-of-class format, rather than completing certain DDL tasks in-class for pair/group work, as illustrated by the following quote.

> [Student A] I thought the DDL activities were useful, but I think although we did it in class I think it would have also been nice to do this more at home, so we would have more time to explore it ourselves. I think it's more effective if we do it outside of class then bring in our results and go through the answers in class.

However, both students mentioned that more in-class training on some of the specific functions might also have been advisable. There was still a perceived need by some for a more 'guided' approach (following Perez-Parades et al.'s 2011 DDL study) for certain functions of the corpus platform, such as reading concordances or understanding collocation information.

> [Student A] I think the different shortcuts and flexibility of the search terms using the corpus is a convenient function, but these could be reinforced in class a little more, just so we can remember I guess. It's quite a new system.

Both students also commented on the selection of the DDL tasks we had made. The sequencing and selection of target items/functions for the corpus tasks was intended to complement the other pre-existing non-corpus based tasks designed around a particular problem or situation that the students would encounter as novice thesis writers, following Aston (1995) and Hafner and Candlin (2007). Student A, however, felt that the corpus tasks should focus on resolving common language-specific difficulties from the outset, so as to reinforce the importance and value of the entire exercise. This was an opinion also shared by Student B.

> [Student A] I know some of the tasks, they are supposed to be easy to introduce people into using the corpus, but if you ask us to search for relatively easy terms like 'I' or 'my' and then we get the results, it doesn't register in our heads how useful it can be, but if you give us more complicated terms to look up, like things we might not know how to express in a sentence properly, then maybe it could give us a better idea into how useful it all is.
>
> [Student B] The tasks could have focused on some key terms from the year before, or professional terms or more difficult action words [sic]. You know, the common problems that we have trouble with.

Crucially, our findings in Chapter 6 regarding the issue of dropout from the DDL activities for some students, and a lack of continued corpus use upon completion of the taught component of the course, warrant serious consideration. Despite the encouraging evidence of sustained and creative corpus use from some students during the taught period, clearly not all students engaged with the corpus, the activities, or the platform. Previous studies focusing on Chinese students of English have suggested that the issue could be a general lack of learner autonomy resulting from a secondary education experience where the teacher is the central source of knowledge and where there is always a 'right' answer for any question (Luo, 2016). Learner autonomy and the willingness to explore alternative hypotheses are crucial pre-requisites (and eventual goals) of the DDL approach, yet wrestling students away from their translation websites is still a lot to ask, as shown in this comment from a student following DDL instruction.

> I like Baidu [a popular Chinese search portal] better since I can usually get a direct answer about how to correct errors by simply typing in an expression or a sentence. (Luo, 2016: p. 10)

This was also the case for the students we interviewed. When asked about the advantages of corpora over other alternatives, both students mentioned that Google appeared to be their primary language reference resource (Student B: "*It's just a reflex, my fingers are just adapted to pressing Google*"). Students' use of search engines has become so normalised (Bax, 2011) that the purely linguistic or statistical results offered via our corpus platform may be insufficient or at least out of tune with students' expectations of what you can *do* with the data.

> [Student B] For me the corpus platform was quite useful but in the future it would be useful to incorporate a link to Pubmed or a similar platform to help us link or somehow connect the corpus findings to relevant journal papers. Kind of like a search engine, using key search terms for an article which might help us to find similar topics to study on.

Accessibility was also considered a factor. Our platform was offered via the Moodle® LMS, but to access this requires a log-in to the university's website, then a click through to the Dentistry ED course Moodle site, then an additional click through to the corpus platform. Students felt this was a few steps too far.

> [Student A] The platform itself is quite efficient, you just type in a word and it shows the results. However, we need a way to make it more convenient, like not having it through Moodle. It should at least be its own site. That would be a factor in making it much more accessible.
>
> [Student B] If more people are going to use it in the future, you should make it an app or dedicated website. For writing I didn't get to use it as often because it just naturally came to me as I wrote – If I had to look it up in the corpus I felt like it was like an extra task to do. I didn't use it much outside of the classroom.

However, both students were impressed with the specificity that a dedicated disciplinary corpus can provide, feeling this was a distinct advantage over general search engines. Such specificity was seen as important for 'writing to learn', at least for novices to the discipline. Interestingly, both students commented that the entire ED course should be scheduled much earlier in the degree programme than its current 5th year, and it is through doing so that the corpus would be more useful.

> [Student A] You can look at it both ways, when generating ideas for a project, a wider spectrum is better. Later down the road, when you know what you are doing, what your project is, then more specific searches with the corpus are probably more helpful, that could really help with our writing, getting the proper patterns and sentence structures that we really need.

> [Student B] Searching the corpus definitely helps you get a better idea of what is important. One of the first words we typed in was tooth, and this showed the common words associated with tooth, and that's actually quite interesting because the first result that popped up was 'tooth wear'. That's one of the most common pathologies that you see in dentistry, so I guess like from this you can indirectly deduce the common concerns that people would have dentistry.
>
> [Student A] I agree, it's more useful for junior students, if they could see what the common search terms were, they could get a better idea about what concepts are more widely searched by the public and what concerns the public have.

In summary, specificity is the factor viewed most positively by the students in terms of their overall appraisal of our DDL approach. Issues with accessibility, the fully normalised use of other reference resources (e.g. Google), and an expectation that the corpus should only be used to resolve language issues appear to be the main factors negatively influencing student uptake of DDL in this context.

7.2.2 ESAP tutors' perceptions of DDL

Aside from the second author of this book, two other ESAP teachers taught on the ED course in question during the experimental period. We interviewed them informally after the course to gauge their perceptions of the effectiveness of the corpus platform and DDL activities regarding improvements to students' motivation, knowledge of disciplinary language, and engagement with the corpus platform. We also asked the teachers if they were comfortable using the corpus platform during in-class activities and whether they had any recommendations for future improvements.

The two ESAP teachers' overall impression of the DDL component of the course was that it was "very interesting", and "had the potential of making the overall experience more rewarding for both teachers and students". Concerning the corpus tasks developed for the ED course, Teacher A observed that his students managed to complete all tasks in class, and in general he found the tasks interesting and useful. However, Teacher B noted the first task on self-mention (i.e. use of 'I' and 'we') might not be that interesting for students as the topic was rather straightforward and easy for these dentistry students.

> [Teacher A] I did manage to get all my students to complete all corpus tasks in class. I found corpus very useful and I like teaching these students in this course.
> [Teacher B] I think some students might see the corpus as useful, but in general my view is that my students are quite negative towards the corpus tasks. The problem is that more of my students are native or near native, and they would might not find the tasks on using 'I', or tenses that interesting or useful.

The mixed feelings regarding the teacher's perception of the corpus tasks are based on the mixed language abilities of their respective students. Teachers of mixed ability classes may find it more difficult to cater to different English learning needs and to accommodate the different learning styles of their students. One possible solution to this problem is to foster cooperation between students of mixed abilities in class through specific DDL activities that emphasise the need for teamwork. Teachers can pair stronger students with less proficient students and involve both in the group discussion of corpus tasks to ensure maximum participation. The stronger students can take on the role of a helper or mentor, to facilitate and scaffold the corpus consultation to generate a more positive learning environment for weaker learners, in line with a sociocultural approach to language acquisition.

As for the corpus platform, both teachers felt that it functioned perfectly, as well as served as an effective channel for students to learn about the differences between learner and expert writing in the dentistry domain. They commented that students rarely asked for help regarding technical issues, or when interpreting the data. Both teachers also felt that getting the dentistry students to use a corpus in this ED course was a good professional development experience, as it was the first course they had taught on that applied the use of a corpus within the curriculum.

> [Teacher A] I enjoy the corpus very much. I'm so glad I can use it in a disciplinary-specific course here.
>
> [Teacher B] This is the very first time for me to use a corpus to teach an ED course here. I found it very meaningful and rewarding for me, and I expect what is done on this course can be transferred to teaching other ED courses.

When asked for any suggestions to improve the corpus tasks or the corpus platform, both teachers felt the need for enabling dentistry students to transfer what they had learned in the activities directly into their writing.

> [Teacher B] I think the corpus is good, but we need to ensure our students are using the corpus to actually help with their writing. To be honest, I haven't directly seen the transfer of what they have been learning to their writing. There seems to have a gap, you know, and we need to think about how to deal with that.

Both teachers believed that it was important to get students to understand the value of the corpus for their writing. To do so, it was suggested by both teachers that the corpus could be introduced to students as early as possible, such as in the first or second session of the course. In this way, students would be introduced to the benefits and advantages of corpora from the outset, potentially increasing motivation to use the corpus for the rest of the course. The teachers also felt the corpus tasks in the course booklet could be moved online, where students could receive instant feedback via the Moodle platform, emphasizing the key role in fostering meaningful interaction between student and instructional materials (Buchanan, 2000). Detailed online feedback could be provided so that upon completion of a corpus task, students can receive instant feedback on correct answers, an explanation for any incorrect answer, or tips for making a more sensible corpus search for the task. This kind of feedback could be acted upon by students to improve their corpus queries, and further promote students' autonomous learning.

7.2.3 Disciplinary tutor's perceptions of DDL

Finally, we interviewed a key disciplinary tutor on their perceptions of the corpus platform and DDL. Professor X is the programme coordinator for the dentistry degree programme and the CHP capstone project. Unlike some of the disciplinary tutors in Hyland (2013a, 2013b), Professor X is quite clear about the importance of language instruction for success in the discipline. They are also very enthusiastic about the ongoing partnership between ESAP professionals and disciplinary tutors as part of English-in-the-discipline.

> Increasingly we expect students to be involved in activities of communication, with patients, staff and the community. [...] One of the problems we have had in the past, because we are doing this through English which is not necessarily their first language, so one of the values of that is to get them to understand not only which words are being used in scientific publications but also the context the words are used in. Language is key to the communication and how they describe it. One of the challenges is that what we do is quite quantitative, which is something quite new for students. It's really the language of science in describing that, both descriptively and analytically.
>
> The CHP is one of the largest bodies of work they do, and since we have had the collaboration the language really has improved, quite dramatically. [As a result of ED] We see a much more clear and concise scientific approach to it in terms of what is the rationale for the project and the importance of what they find, and this has now become more concise and clear and also much less subjective.

When questioned about the role of the corpus and DDL within ED provision, Professor X highlighted the benefits to autonomy DDL can provide in the group project context of the CHP, as well as the specificity afforded via the use of a disciplinary corpus. They also mentioned the benefits afforded through student consultation with both professional and learner corpora in the course materials. The professor's focus on the importance of context in learning about disciplinary language also extends to their perceptions of the functionality of the corpus platform.

> Our students vary, and their language skills are different, but certainly the corpus gives students the ability within the group that if they themselves want to check things on for themselves independent from class they have the ability to do so. Students are also less likely to go back to the kind of things we will have used, like the dictionary, and I think the corpus is giving us information very specific to the project at hand.
>
> You've got the learner corpus which gives them an example of the words and the context they are used, and that's also supported by the professional corpus which is aligned to a key publication, one of the most common journals they might get at the undergraduate level with other journals being quite technical. However, it is interesting that the learner corpus gets searched more, its more valuable and that is because it fits more with the style of the project – it's not necessarily a research article, it's about how they have delivered a service.
>
> Regarding the platform] Two things come to mind: I like the fact you can search for the words and see the context, how the word is used; and I thought the aspect of collocation where you can visualise what words are used close to it was very interesting, you aren't going to see that from online dictionaries.

When asked about the students' lack of corpus use beyond the project, the professor acknowledged the need to increase accessibility through the development of a mobile app, but did note that a number of students return to the university upon graduation to take on postgraduate studies. It would therefore be interesting to see how many returning graduates use the corpus to complete their postgraduate assignments, and other disciplinary tutors responsible for postgraduates should be made aware of the corpus. Finally, the professor provided very positive comments about the value of DDL and the corpus platform for the promotion of 'writing-to-learn'.

> Oral communication with patients is one thing, that's very much in lay terminology at times, but when writing the report they are really getting that 'scientific' communication. Clearly, not all of them or not many of them might not continue in that field, but even as practicing dentists they will be actively involved in continuing learning and interpreting scientific discourse. The corpus should definitely help them to do this – it's a key skill to have, that's how you can be actively involved [as a professional], interpreting [research] findings, and then making the science yourself.

7.3 What is left to do?

While we feel this volume has provided a solid practical foundation for ESAP professionals and corpus linguists who wish to conduct further research into disciplinary writing and DDL, there are still a number of developments that we have, as yet, been unable to incorporate. Here, we discuss a number of opportunities that we would like to pursue in the not-too-distant future.

One criticism levelled at corpus-based ESAP work is that most corpora and corpus tasks are still largely focused on 'low-level' phenomena involving grammar and lexis, while corpora that facilitate analysis of 'higher-level' phenomena at the discourse or genre level are still relatively rare (Boulton, Carter-Thomas & Jolivet, 2012: p. 3). While we were able to build a set of course materials that allowed for both 'low level' and 'higher level' analysis through a mix of corpus tasks and non-corpus based activities on larger sections of text (as seen in other studies such as Charles, 2007), the corpus tasks themselves were necessarily focused on grammar and disciplinary lexis, and students were unable to use the corpus to investigate spans of text larger than the concordance line. One reason for this design choice is that despite having the technical ability to display, say, the paragraph from which a given concordance result was found, we then run the risk of violating our university's ethics procedures in terms of the storage and dissemination of copyright materials. Our university's ethics board allowed for data from the professional and learner corpora shown in Chapter 3 to be used for the online corpus platform in Chapter 5, but only on the condition that concordance lines, rather than larger segments of text, could be displayed to students. While university ethics panels differ globally in their understanding of corpus research and copyright issues, within the context of this volume, we were unable to display the amount of information (e.g. a paragraph, a section, or even a full text) that would be required for 'higher level' corpus-based analysis.

However, in the theoretical event that copyright/ethics are not issues for the researcher or teacher, there are promising developments in the field that might allow for meaningful corpus-based analysis of 'higher level' discourse elements. One such example is found in Thomas (2015), which focuses on how the study of collocation often requires more information about the context of use and suggests the incorporation of a feature that he calls 'collocation plus' or C+. C+ collocations are 'extended' collocations that can be used to generate so-called "topic trails" (p. 99) of key nouns and their verb collocates that eventually constitute the 'aboutness' of the text. This is deemed particularly useful for polysemous targets, given the disambiguation provided by the context, and could potentially help our students overcome some of the issues related to polysemy uncovered in the findings for case reports in Chapter 4. We are also beginning to see the use of genre annotated corpora in the language classroom, most recently seen in Cotos, Link and Huffman (2017) as part of their purpose-built *Research Writing Tutor* (RWT) platform. This platform combines a corpus annotated for rhetorical composition including moves/steps (e.g. Swales, 1990) with its own concordancer, together with video lectures, readings, and an automated feedback function. Obviously, this platform is the current state-of-the-art in terms of facilitating DDL for L2 writing at the bottom-up and top-down levels and could lead to measurable gains in genre awareness. Ethics issues non-withstanding, future research in this area does appear to point towards the necessity for an integrated approach to DDL provision of the type seen in Cotos et al's study if we are to do all we can for corpus-based DDL to succeed in disciplinary writing contexts.

However, despite ongoing efforts, the issue of feedback on L2 writing is one that is still problematic for DDL, as shown in Crosthwaite (2017). As yet, we do not have a DDL-specific approach to written corrective feedback at the lexico-grammatical level, let alone the discourse level, and it is unclear whether the automated feedback provided in Cotos et al.'s RMT is suitable for subsequent corpus queries. The feedback required for meaningful DDL to occur should be neither too vague for students to generate appropriate corpus queries on the one hand, nor so informative that it negates the need for students to query the corpus. DDL studies have historically varied in the form of feedback provided, making it difficult to generalise the results of one study to another. The first author is currently involved in an experimental project in Australia to determine which feedback form is most conducive to DDL error resolution in L2 writing, both generally and specific to particular error types, and with the variables ranging from highlighting some of the context around an error, highlighting and locating the error, highlighting and providing an error code, and highlighting with indirect feedback. The results of this research will be made available in the near future.

Another area for investigation is that of the need for studies investigating the longitudinal effects of corpora and DDL on writing/language development in the medium to long term (Boulton, 2011; Luo, 2016). Most DDL studies typically last for up to a semester, meaning that claims regarding DDL's impact on writing development (e.g. accuracy, complexity, fluency), while valid within the context of individual studies, need to be supported with further evidence from longer term studies. Again, this work is now underway, headed by the first author in a project at the University of Queensland which aims to build a longitudinal corpus of L1 and L2 student writing across the university's Bachelor of Arts program across the three-year duration of the degree. Students on the program are to be trained in their first semester to use the BAWE corpus for resolving language issues through a short private online course (Crosthwaite, 2018). After the first year, the first author intends to analyse the students' data to identify individuals who may be experiencing a particular difficulty in their writing (e.g. overusing boosters when making claims). These selected students will then take remedial lectures (or 'targeted interventions') focusing on these specific issues, in what might presumably be the first example of corpus-based *data-driven teaching* in the DDL literature – where learner corpus data is used to determine the specific language issues these particular students are struggling with, before teaching them how to overcome them. Their progress will continue to be monitored via corpus analysis of their written production throughout the lifespan of their degree, charting their longitudinal development as writers for the Arts. Data collection is ongoing.

7.4 Closing comments

This volume is the very first monograph on the market that deals with a corpus-based analysis of the language of dentistry for the purposes of disciplinary writing. We have successfully shown that corpora can reveal aspects of language that were hitherto vague or invisible. This has changed the way we look at the language of dentistry and resolved the ESAP conundrum the authors were faced with at the outset of the volume. Our corpus-based and corpus-driven insights lay a strong foundation for the kind of curriculum and pedagogical design that truly addresses the actual learning needs of dentistry students, enhancing their academic literacy while mastering the language features of the key genres of dentistry disciplinary writing in tandem with disciplinary content and assessment. It is our hope that this volume results in a re-evaluation of ideas about the teaching and learning of disciplinary writing, and works as a springboard for future research in this vital area of tertiary education.

References

Ädel, A. (2010). Using corpora to teach academic writing: Challenges for the direct approach. In M. C. Campoy-Cubillo, B. Belles-Fortuño, & L. Gea-Valor (Eds.), *Corpus-based approaches to ELT* (pp. 39–55). London: Continuum.

Ädel, A., & Garretson, G. (2006). Citation practices across disciplines: The case of proficient student writing. In M. C. Pérez-Llantada Auría, R. Pló Alastrué, & C. P. Neumann (Eds.), *Academic and professional communication in the 21st century: Genres and rhetoric in the construction of disciplinary knowledge* (pp. 271–280). Zaragoza, Spain: Prensas Universitarias.

Agarwal, A., Xie, B., Vovsha, I., Rambow, O., & Passonneau, R. (2011, June). Sentiment analysis of twitter data. In *Proceedings of the workshop on languages in social media* (pp. 30–38). Stroudsburg, PA: Association for Computational Linguistics.

Aldabe, I. (2011). *Automatic exercise generation based on corpora and natural language processing techniques* (Unpublished doctoral dissertation). Euskal Herriko Unibertsitatea (University of the Basque Country), San Sebastian, Basque Country.

Alexopoulou, T., Michel, M., Murakami, A., & Meurers, D. (2017). Task effects on linguistic complexity and accuracy: A large-scale learner corpus analysis employing natural language processing techniques. *Language Learning*, 67(S1), 180–208. https://doi.org/10.1111/lang.12232

Altman, D., & Mascarenhas, A. K. (2016). New competencies for the 21st century dental public health specialist. *Journal of Public Health Dentistry*, 76(s18–s28). https://doi.org/10.1111/jphd.12190

Aluthman, E. S. (2017). The impact of the data-driven learning approach on ESL writers' citation patterns. *International Journal of English Linguistics*, 7(6), 109–122. https://doi.org/10.5539/ijel.v7n6p109

Amdur, R., Kirwan, J., & Morris C. (2010). Use of the passive voice in medical journal articles. *American Medical Writers Association Journal*, 25(3), 98–110.

Anthony, L. (2014). *AntConc* (version 3.4.4). [Computer Software]. Tokyo, Japan: Waseda University. Available from <http://www.laurenceanthony.net/software>

Anthony, L. (2016). Introducing corpora and corpus tools into the technical writing classroom through data-driven learning. In J. Flowerdew & T. Costley (Eds.), *Discipline specific writing* (pp. 162–180). London: Routledge.

Anthony, L. (2017a). Introducing corpora and corpus tools into the technical writing classroom through data-driven learning (DDL). In J. Flowerdew & T. Costley (Eds.), *Discipline-specific writing: Theory into practice* (pp. 162–180). London: Routledge.

Anthony, L. (2017b). *AntFileConverter* (version 1.2.1) [Computer Software]. Tokyo, Japan: Waseda University. Available from <http://www.laurenceanthony.net/software>

Anthony, L. (2018). Introduction. In L. Anthony (Ed.), *Introducing English for Specific Purposes* (pp. 1–6). New York, NY: Routledge.

Applebee, A. (1996). *Curriculum as conversation: Transforming traditions of teaching and learning*. Chicago, IL: University of Chicago Press.

Aston, G. (1995). Corpora in language pedagogy: matching theory and practice. In G. Cook & B. Seidlhofer (Eds.), *Principles and practice in applied linguistics* (pp. 257–270). Oxford: Oxford University Press.

Athar, A. (2011, June). Sentiment analysis of citations using sentence structure-based features. In *Proceedings of the ACL 2011 student session* (pp. 81–87). Stroudsburg, PA: Association for Computational Linguistics.

Aull, L. L., & Lancaster, Z. (2014). Linguistic markers of stance in early and advanced academic writing: A corpus-based comparison. *Written Communication*, 31, 151–183. https://doi.org/10.1177/0741088314527055

Baisa, V., & Suchomel, V. (2014, December). Skell: Web interface for english language learning. In A. Horák & P. Rychlý (Eds.), *Eighth Workshop on Recent Advances in Slavonic Natural Language Processing, RASLAN 2014* (pp. 63–70). Brno: Tribun EU.

Barrón-Cedeño, A., Vila, M., Martí, M. A., & Rosso, P. (2013). Plagiarism meets paraphrasing: Insights for the next generation in automatic plagiarism detection. *Computational Linguistics*, 39(4), 917–947. https://doi.org/10.1162/COLI_a_00153

Basturkmen, H. (2012). A genre-based investigation of discussion sections of research articles in dentistry and disciplinary variation. *Journal of English for Academic Purposes*, 11(2), 134–144. https://doi.org/10.1016/j.jeap.2011.10.004

Bax, S. (2011). Normalisation revisited: The effective use of technology in language education. *International Journal of Computer-Assisted Language Learning and Teaching (IJCALLT)*, 1(2), 1–15. https://doi.org/10.4018/ijcallt.2011040101

Bazerman, C. (2002). Genre and identity: Citizenship in the age of the internet and the age of global capitalism. In R. Coe, L. Lingard, & T. Teslenko (Eds.), *The rhetoric and ideology of genre* (pp. 13–37). Cresskill, NJ: Hampton Press.

Bernardini, S. (2001). Corpora in the classroom: An overview and some reflections on future developments. In J. Sinclair (Ed.), *How to use corpora in language teaching* (pp. 15–36). Amsterdam: John Benjamins.

Biber, D. (1988). *Variation across speech and writing*. Cambridge: Cambridge University Press. https://doi.org/10.1017/CBO9780511621024

Biber, D. (1989). A typology of English texts. *Linguistics*, 27(1), 3–43. https://doi.org/10.1515/ling.1989.27.1.3

Biber, D. (1994). An analytical framework for register studies. In D. Biber & E. Finegan (Eds.), *Sociolinguistic perspectives on register* (pp. 31–56). Oxford: Oxford University Press.

Biber, D. (1995). *Dimensions of register variation: A cross-linguistic comparison*. Cambridge: Cambridge University Press. https://doi.org/10.1017/CBO9780511519871

Biber, D. (2006a). *University language: A corpus-based study of spoken and written registers*. Amsterdam: John Benjamins. https://doi.org/10.1075/scl.23

Biber, D. (2006b). Stance in spoken and written university registers. *Journal of English for Academic Purposes*, 5(2), 97–116. https://doi.org/10.1016/j.jeap.2006.05.001

Biber, D., & Conrad, S. (2009). *Register, genre, and style*. Cambridge: Cambridge University Press. https://doi.org/10.1017/CBO9780511814358

Biber, D., & Finegan, E. (1994). Intra-textual variation within medical research articles. In J. Aarts (Ed.), *Corpus-based research into language* (pp. 201–222). Amsterdam: Rodopi.

Biber, D., & Gray, B. (2010). Challenging stereotypes about academic writing: Complexity, elaboration, explicitness. *Journal of English for Academic Purposes*, 9(1), 2–20. https://doi.org/10.1016/j.jeap.2010.01.001

Biber, D., & Gray, B. (2013). Being specific about historical change: The influence of sub-register. *Journal of English Linguistics*, 41(2), 104–134. https://doi.org/10.1177/0075424212472509

Biber, D., & Gray, B. (2016). *Grammatical complexity in academic English: Linguistic change in writing*. Cambridge: Cambridge University Press. https://doi.org/10.1017/CBO9780511920776

Biber, D., & Kurjian, J. (2007). Towards a taxonomy of web registers and text types: A multi-dimensional analysis. *Language and Computers*, 59, 109.

Birch-Becaas, S., & Cooke, R. (2012). Raising collective awareness of rhetorical strategies: Using an online writing tool to demonstrative discourse moves in the ESP classroom. In A. Boulton, S. Carter-Thomas, & E. Rowley-Jolivet (Eds.), *Corpus-informed research and learning in ESP: Issues and applications* (pp. 239–260). Amsterdam: John Benjamins. https://doi.org/10.1075/scl.52.10bir

Bley-Vroman, R. (1989). What is the logical problem of foreign language learning? In S. M. Gass & J. Schachter (Eds.), *Linguistic perspectives on second language acquisition* (pp. 41–68) New York, NY: Cambridge University Press. https://doi.org/10.1017/CBO9781139524544.005

Blue, G. M. (1988). Individualising academic writing tuition. In P. Robinson (Ed.), *Academic writing: Process and product*. Oxford: Modern English Publications.

Boulton, A. (2011). Data-driven learning: The perpetual enigma. In S. Goźdź-Roszkowski (Ed.), *Explorations across languages and corpora* (pp. 563–580). Frankfurt: Peter Lang.

Boulton, A. (2015). Applying data-driven learning to the web. In A. Lénko-Szymánska & A. Boulton (Eds.), *Multiple affordances of language corpora for data-driven learning* (pp. 267–295). Amsterdam: John Benjamins.

Boulton, A. (2012). Corpus consultation for ESP: A review of empirical research. In A. Boulton, S. Carter-Thomas, & E. Rowley-Jolivet (Eds.), *Corpus-informed research and learning in ESP: Issues and applications* (pp. 261–292). Amsterdam: John Benjamins. https://doi.org/10.1075/scl.52.11bou

Boulton, A., Carter-Thomas, S., & Rowley-Jolivet, E. (Eds.). (2012). *Corpus-informed research and learning in ESP: Issues and applications*. Amsterdam: John Benjamins. https://doi.org/10.1075/scl.52

Boulton, A., & Cobb, T. (2017). Corpus use in language learning: A meta-analysis. *Language Learning*, 67(2), 348–393. https://doi.org/10.1111/lang.12224

Brezina, V. (2018). *Statistics in corpus linguistics: A practical guide*. Cambridge: Cambridge University Press.

Browne, M. W., & Cudeck, R. (1992). Alternative ways of assessing model fit. *Sociological Methods & Research*, 21(2), 230–258. https://doi.org/10.1177/0049124192021002005

Buchanan, T. (2000). The efficacy of a World-Wide Web mediated formative assessment. *Journal of Computer Assisted Learning*, 16, 193–200. https://doi.org/10.1046/j.1365-2729.2000.00132.x

Carlson, D. M. (2000). A corpus-linguistic investigation of dental English. *Journal of Dental Education*, 64(4), 283–293.

Carter, R. A., & McCarthy, M. J. (1995). Grammar and the spoken language. *Applied Linguistics*, 16, 141–158.

Cattell, R. B. (1966). The scree test for the number of factors. *Multivariate Behavioral Research*, 1(2), 245–276. https://doi.org/10.1207/s15327906mbr0102_10

Chen, M., & Flowerdew, J. (2018). Introducing data-driven learning to PhD students for research writing purposes: A territory-wide project in Hong Kong. *English for Specific Purposes*, 50, 97–112. https://doi.org/10.1016/j.esp.2017.11.004

Chambers, A. (2007). Popularising corpus consultation by language learners and teachers. In E. Hidalgo, L. Quereda, & J. Santana (Eds.), *Corpora in the foreign language classroom* (pp. 3–16). Amsterdam: Rodopi. https://doi.org/10.1163/9789401203906_002

Chambers, A., & O'Sullivan, I. (2004). Corpus consultation and advanced learners' writing skills in French. *ReCALL*, 16, 158–172. https://doi.org/10.1017/S0958344004001211

Charles, M. (2007). Reconciling top-down and bottom-up approaches to graduate writing: Using a corpus to teach rhetorical functions. *Journal of English for Academic Purposes*, 6(4), 289–302. https://doi.org/10.1016/j.jeap.2007.09.009

Charles, M. (2014). Getting the corpus habit: EAP students' long-term use of personal corpora. *English for Specific Purposes*, 35(1), 30–40. https://doi.org/10.1016/j.esp.2013.11.004

Charles, M. (2015). Same task, different corpus: The role of personal corpora in EAP classes. In A. Lénko-Szymánska & A. Boulton (Eds.), *Multiple affordances of language corpora for data-driven learning* (pp. 131–153). Amsterdam: John Benjamins.

Chun, C. (2017). Critical literacy writing in ESP: Perspectives and approaches. In J. Flowerdew & T. Costley (Eds.), *Discipline-specific writing: Theory into practice* (pp. 181–195). London: Routledge.

Christie, H., Tett, L., Cree, V. E., Hounsell, J., & McCune, V. (2008). 'A real rollercoaster of confidence and emotions': Learning to be a university student. *Studies in Higher Education*, 33(5), 567–581. https://doi.org/10.1080/03075070802373040

Cobb, T., & Boulton, A. (2015). Classroom applications of corpus analysis. In D. Biber & R. Reppen (Eds.), *Cambridge handbook of English corpus linguistics* (pp. 478–497). Cambridge: Cambridge University Press. https://doi.org/10.1017/CBO9781139764377.027

Cohen, A. M., & Hersh, W. R. (2005). A survey of current work in biomedical text mining. *Briefings in Bioinformatics*, 6(1), 57–71. https://doi.org/10.1093/bib/6.1.57

Cohen, J. (1988). *Statistical power analysis for the behavioral sciences* (2nd ed.). Hillsdale, NJ: Lawrence Erlbaum Associates.

Cortes, V. (2004). Lexical bundles in published and student disciplinary writing: Examples from history and biology. *English for Specific Purposes*, 23(4), 397–423. https://doi.org/10.1016/j.esp.2003.12.001

Cortes, V. (2007). Genre and corpora in the English for academic writing class. *ORTESOL Journal*, 25, 9–16.

Cortes, V., & Csomay, E. (Eds.). (2015). *Corpus-based research in applied linguistics: Studies in honor of Doug Biber*. Amsterdam: John Benjamins. https://doi.org/10.1075/scl.66

Cotos, E. (2014). Enhancing writing pedagogy with learner corpus data. *ReCALL*, 26(2), 202–224. https://doi.org/10.1017/S0958344014000019

Cotos, E., Link, S., & Huffman, S. (2017). Effects of technology on genre learning. *Language Learning & Technology*, 21(3), 104–130.

Coxhead, A. (2000). A new academic word list. *TESOL Quarterly*, 34(2), 213–238. https://doi.org/10.2307/3587951

Coxhead, A., & Nation, P. (2001). The specialised vocabulary of English for academic purposes. In J. Flowerdew & M. Peacock (Eds.), *Research perspectives on English for academic purposes* (pp. 252–267). Cambridge: Cambridge University Press. https://doi.org/10.1017/CBO9781139524766.020

Crawford, J. M., Adami, G., Johnson, B. R., Knight, G. W., Knoernschild, K., Obrez, A., Patson, P., Punwani, I., Zaki, A. & Licari, F. W. (2007). Curriculum restructuring at a North American dental school: rationale for change. *Journal of Dental Education*, 71(4), 524–531.

Crossley, S. A., Kyle, K., & McNamara, D. S. (2016). The tool for the automatic analysis of text cohesion (TAACO): Automatic assessment of local, global, and text cohesion. *Behavior Research Methods*, 48(4), 1227–1237. https://doi.org/10.3758/s13428-015-0651-7

Crossley, S. A., Kyle, K., & McNamara, D. S. (2017). Sentiment analysis and social cognition engine (SEANCE): An automatic tool for sentiment, social cognition, and social-order analysis. *Behavior Research Methods*, 49(3), 803–821. https://doi.org/10.3758/s13428-016-0743-z

Crossley, S., Russell, D., Kyle, K., & Römer, U. (2017). Applying natural language processing tools to a student academic writing corpus: How large are disciplinary differences across science and engineering fields? *Journal of Writing Analytics*, 1, 48–81.

Crossley, S., Kyle, K. & Romer, U. (2019). Examining lexical and cohesion differences in discipline-specific writing using multi-dimensional analysis. In Tony Berber Sardinha & Marcia Veirano Pinto (eds.) *Multi-Dimensional Analysis: Research Methods and Current Issues* (pp. 189–216). London, UK: Bloomsbury.

Crosthwaite, P. (2016). A longitudinal multidimensional analysis of EAP writing: Determining EAP course effectiveness. *Journal of English for Academic Purposes*, 22, 166–178. https://doi.org/10.1016/j.jeap.2016.04.005

Crosthwaite, P. (2017). Retesting the limits of data-driven learning: Feedback and error correction. *Computer Assisted Language Learning*, 30(6), 447–473. https://doi.org/10.1080/09588221.2017.1312462

Crosthwaite, P. (2018, June 8). Scaling up DDL: Challenges of bringing DDL to an online SPOC format. Video conference paper presented at *2nd BAAL Corpus Linguistics SIG event 2018: New Directions in DDL*. Centre for Academic Writing, Coventry University, UK.

Crosthwaite, P., Cheung, L., & Jiang, F. K. (2017). Writing with attitude: Stance expression in learner and professional dentistry research reports. *English for Specific Purposes*, 46, 107–123. https://doi.org/10.1016/j.esp.2017.02.001

Crosthwaite, P., & Jiang, K. (2017). Does EAP affect written L2 academic stance? A longitudinal learner corpus study. *System*, 69, 92–107. https://doi.org/10.1016/j.system.2017.06.010

Crosthwaite, P., Wong, L. L. C., & Cheung, O. W. (2019). Characterising postgraduate students' corpus query and usage patterns for disciplinary data-driven learning. *ReCALL*, online ahead of print. https://doi.org/10.1017/S0958344019000077

Cumming, A. (1990). Metalinguistic and ideational thinking in second language composing. *Written Communication*, 7, 482–511. https://doi.org/10.1177/0741088390007004003

Dagneux, E., Denness, S., & Granger, S. (1998). Computer-aided error analysis. *System*, 26, 163–174. https://doi.org/10.1016/S0346-251X(98)00001-3

Dahl, T., (2004). Textual metadiscourse in research articles: A marker of national culture or of academic discipline? *Journal of Pragmatics*, 36, 1807–1825. https://doi.org/10.1016/j.pragma.2004.05.004

Davies, M. (2004). *BYU-BNC. Based on the British National Corpus from Oxford University Press.* Available online at <http://corpus.byu.edu/bnc>

Ding, D. (1998). Rationality reborn: Historical roots of the passive voice in scientific discourse. In J. T. Battalio (Ed.), *Essays in the study of scientific discourse: Methods, practice, and pedagogy* (pp. 117–135). Stamford, CT: Ablex.

Dittmar, N. (2010). Register. In M. Fried, J. A. Östman, & J. Verschueren (Eds.), *Variation and change: Pragmatic perspectives* (pp. 221–233). Amsterdam: John Benjamins. https://doi.org/10.1075/hoph.6.16dit

Dorgeloh, H. (2016). The interrelationship of register and genre in medical discourse. In C. Schubert & C. Sanchez-Stockhammer (Eds.), *Variational text linguistics: Revisiting register in English* (pp. 42–66). Berlin: De Gruyter. https://doi.org/10.1515/9783110443554-004

Dorgeloh, H., & Wanner, A. (2010). *Syntactic variation and genre*. Berlin: De Gruyter. https://doi.org/10.1515/9783110226485

Durrant, P. (2017). Lexical bundles and disciplinary variation in university students' writing: Mapping the territories. *Applied Linguistics* 38(2), 165–193. https://doi.org/10.1093/applin/amv011

Evans, S. (2011). Hong Kong English and the professional world. *World Englishes*, 30(3), 293–316. https://doi.org/10.1111/j.1467-971X.2011.01655.x

Evans, S., & Green, C. (2007). Why EAP is necessary: A survey of Hong Kong tertiary students. *Journal of English for Academic Purposes*, 6(1), 3–17. https://doi.org/10.1016/j.jeap.2006.11.005

Evans, S., & Morrison, B. (2011). The first term at university: Implications for EAP. *English Language Teaching Journal*, 65(4), 376–386. https://doi.org/10.1093/elt/ccq072

Evert, S. (2018, June). The hermeneutic cyborg. Conference abstract for *13th Annual Sinclair Open Lecture*, June 25th, University of Birmingham, UK.

Faculty of Dentistry, The University of Hong Kong. (2015). Regulations for the Degree of Bachelor of Dental Surgery (BDS). Retrieved from <http://facdent.hku.hk/learning/ug_info/BDS%206-Year%20Regs%20and%20Sylls%202015-16-Dec2015.pdf>

Feldman, R., & Sanger, J. (2007). *The text mining handbook: Advanced approaches in analyzing unstructured data.* Cambridge: Cambridge University Press.

Ferguson, G. (1997). Teacher education and LSP: The role of specialised knowledge. In R. Howard & G. Brown (Eds.), *Teacher education for Languages for Specific Purposes* (pp. 80–89). Clevedon: Multilingual Matters.

Flowerdew, J. (2016). English for Specific Academic Purposes: Making the case. *Writing and Pedagogy*, 8(1), 5–32. https://doi.org/10.1558/wap.v8i1.30051

Flowerdew, J., & Costley (Eds.). (2017). *Discipline-specific writing: Theory into practice.* London: Routledge.

Flowerdew, L. (2015). Data-driven learning and language learning theories: Wither the twain shall meet. In A. Lénko-Szymánska & A. Boulton (Eds.), *Multiple affordances of language corpora for data-driven learning* (pp. 15–36). Amsterdam: John Benjamins.

Frankenberg-Garcia, A. (2005). A peek into what today's language learners as researchers actually do. *International Journal of Lexicography*, 18, 335–355. https://doi.org/10.1093/ijl/eci015

Friginal, E., & Hardy, J. (2014). Conducting Biber's multi-dimensional analysis using SPSS. In T. Berber Sardinha & M. Veirano Pinto (Eds.), *Multi-dimensional analysis: 25 years on* (pp. 297–316). Amsterdam: John Benjamins. https://doi.org/10.1075/scl.60.10fri

Fryer, D. L. (2013). Exploring the dialogism of academic discourse: Heteroglossic engagement in medical research articles. In G. Andersen & K. Bech (Eds.), *English corpus linguistics: Variation in time, space and genre: Selected papers from International Computer Archive of Modern and Medieval English (ICAME)* (pp. 183–207). Leiden: Brill.

Fuentes, A. C. (2017). Form-focused data-driven learning for grammar development in ESP contexts. *Revista de Lenguas para Fines Específicos*, 23(1), 12–30.

Gaskell, D., & Cobb, T. (2004). Can learners use concordance feedback for writing errors? *System*, 32, 301–319. https://doi.org/10.1016/j.system.2004.04.001

Gardner, S., Nesi, H., & Biber, D. (2018). Discipline, level, genre: Integrating situational perspectives in a new MD analysis of university student writing. *Applied Linguistics*, 1–30. https://doi.org/10.1093/applin/amy005

Gavioli, L. (2005). *Exploring corpora for ESP learning.* Amsterdam: John Benjamins. https://doi.org/10.1075/scl.21

Gilquin, G. (2000). The integrated contrastive model: Spicing up your data. *Languages in Contrast*, 3, 95–123.

Gopikrishna, V. (2010). A report on case reports. *Journal of Conservative Dentistry*, 13(4), 265–271. https://doi.org/10.4103/0972-0707.73375

Gotti, M., & Salager-Meyer, F. (2006). *Advances in medical discourse analysis: Written and oral contexts.* Berlin: Peter Lang. https://doi.org/10.3726/978-3-0351-0396-0

Granger, S. (1996). From CA to CIA and back: An integrated approach to computerized bilingual and learner corpora. In K. Aijmer, *Languages in contrast. Text-based cross-linguistic studies* (pp. 37–51). Lund: Lund University Press.

Granger, S. (2015). Contrastive interlanguage analysis: A reappraisal. *International Journal of Learner Corpus Research*, 1(1), 7–24. https://doi.org/10.1075/ijlcr.1.1.01gra

Gray, B. (2015). On the complexity of academic writing: Disciplinary variation and structural complexity. In V. Cortes & E. Csomay (Eds.), *Corpus-based research in applied linguistics: Studies in honor of Doug Biber* (pp. 49–78). Amsterdam: John Benjamins. https://doi.org/10.1075/scl.66.03gra

Gross, A. G., & Chesley, P. (2012). Hedging, stance and voice in medical research articles. In K. Hyland & C. S. Guinda (Eds.), *Stance and voice in written academic genres* (pp. 85–100). Houndmills: Palgrave Macmillan. https://doi.org/10.1057/9781137030825_6

Hafner, C. A., & Candlin, C. N. (2007). Corpus tools as an affordance to learning in professional legal education. *Journal of English for Academic Purposes*, 6, 303–318. https://doi.org/10.1016/j.jeap.2007.09.005

Hardy, J. A., & Friginal, E. (2016). Genre variation in student writing: A multi-dimensional analysis. *Journal of English for Academic Purposes*, 22, 119–131. https://doi.org/10.1016/j.jeap.2016.03.002

Hardy, J. A., & Römer, U. (2013). Revealing disciplinary variation in student writing: A multi-dimensional analysis of the Michigan Corpus of Upper-level Student Papers (MICUSP). *Corpora*, 8(2), 183–207. https://doi.org/10.3366/cor.2013.0040

Hawkins, J. A., & Buttery, P. (2010). Criterial features in learner corpora: Theory and illustrations. *English Profile Journal*, 1(1), e5. https://doi.org/10.1017/S2041536210000103

Hernandez, L. M., Rosenstock, L., & Gebbie, K. (Eds.). (2003). *Who will keep the public healthy? Educating public health professionals for the 21st Century*. Washington, DC: National Academies Press.

Herrando-Rodrigo, I. (2010). "If you suffer from … check the Internet": The role of engagement and self-mention devices in medical research articles and electronic popularizations. In R. Lorés-Sanz, P. Mur-Dueñas, & E. Lafuente-Millán (Eds.), *Constructing interpersonality: Multiple perspectives on written academic genres* (pp. 255–274). Newcastle upon Tyne: Cambridge Scholars.

Hinkel, E. (2004). Tense, aspect and the passive voice in L1 and L2 academic texts. *Language Teaching Research*, 8(1), 5–29. https://doi.org/10.1191/1362168804lr132oa

Hirvela, A., Hyland, K., & Manchón, R. M. (2016). Dimensions in L2 writing theory and research: Learning to write and writing to learn. In R. M. Manchón & P. K. Matsuda (Eds.), *Handbook of second and foreign language writing* (pp. 45–64). Berlin: De Gruyter. https://doi.org/10.1515/9781614511335-005

Holmes, J. (1988). Doubt and certainty in ESL textbooks. *Applied Linguistics*, 9(1), 21–44. https://doi.org/10.1093/applin/9.1.21

Holtzman, J. M., Elliot, N., Biber, C. L., & Sanders, R. M. (2005). Computerized assessment of dental student writing skills. *Journal of Dental Education*, 69(2), 285–295.

Hopper, P. J., & Thompson, S. A. (1980). Transitivity in grammar and discourse. *Language*, 56(2), 251–299. https://doi.org/10.1353/lan.1980.0017

Hu, G., & Cao, F. (2015). Disciplinary and paradigmatic influences on interactional metadiscourse in research articles. *English for Specific Purposes*, 39, 12–25. https://doi.org/10.1016/j.esp.2015.03.002

Hu, L. T., & Bentler, P. M. (1998). Fit indices in covariance structure modeling: Sensitivity to underparameterized model misspecification. *Psychological Methods*, 3(4), 424. https://doi.org/10.1037/1082-989X.3.4.424

Hu, M., & Liu, B. (2004). Mining and summarizing customer reviews. In *Proceedings of the Tenth ACM SIGKDD International Conference on Knowledge Discovery and Data Mining* (pp. 168–177). Seattle, WA: ACM.

Hu, N., Bose, I., Koh, N. S., & Liu, L. (2012). Manipulation of online reviews: An analysis of ratings, readability, and sentiments. *Decision Support Systems*, 52(3), 674–684. https://doi.org/10.1016/j.dss.2011.11.002

Huang, Y., Murakami, A., Alexopoulou, T., & Korhonen, A. (2018). Dependency parsing of learner English. *International Journal of Corpus Linguistics*, 23(1), 28–54. https://doi.org/10.1075/ijcl.16080.hua

Hurwitz, B. (2006). Form and representation in clinical case reports. *Literature and Medicine*, 25(2), 216–240.

Hutchinson, T., & Waters, A. (1987). *English for specific purposes: A learning-centred approach*. Cambridge: Cambridge University Press. https://doi.org/10.1017/CBO9780511733031

Hyland, K. (1998). *Hedging in scientific research articles*. Amsterdam: John Benjamins. https://doi.org/10.1075/pbns.54

Hyland, K. (1999). Disciplinary discourses: Writer stance in research articles. In C. Candlin & K. Hyland (Eds), *Writing: Texts, processes and practices* (pp. 99–121). London: Routledge.

Hyland, K. (2000). *Disciplinary discourses: Social interactions in academic writing*. Harlow: Pearson.

Hyland, K. (2004a). *Disciplinary discourses: Social interactions in academic writing*. Ann Arbor, MI: University of Michigan Press.

Hyland, K. (2004b). Disciplinary interactions: Metadiscourse in L2 postgraduate writing. *Journal of Second Language Writing*, 13(2), 133–151. https://doi.org/10.1016/j.jslw.2004.02.001

Hyland, K. (2005). *Metadiscourse: Exploring interaction in writing*. London: Continuum.

Hyland, K. (2007). Genre pedagogy: Language, literacy and L2 writing instruction. *Journal of Second Language Writing*, 16(3), 148–164. https://doi.org/10.1016/j.jslw.2007.07.005

Hyland, K. (2008). As can be seen: Lexical bundles and disciplinary variation. *English for Specific Purposes*, 27(1), 4–21. https://doi.org/10.1016/j.esp.2007.06.001

Hyland, K. (2011). Learning to write. In R. Manchón (ed.) *Learning-to-write and writing-to-learn in an additional language* (pp. 17–36). Amsterdam: John Benjamins. https://doi.org/10.1075/lllt.31.05hyl

Hyland, K. (2012). Undergraduate understandings: Stance and voice in final year reports. In K. Hyland & C. Sancho-Guinda (Eds.), *Stance and voice in written academic genres* (pp. 134–150). Houndmills: Palgrave Macmillan. https://doi.org/10.1057/9781137030825_9

Hyland, K. (2013a). Faculty feedback: Perceptions and practices in L2 disciplinary writing. *Journal of Second Language Writing*, 22, 240–253. https://doi.org/10.1016/j.jslw.2013.03.003

Hyland, K. (2013b). Student perceptions of hidden messages in teacher written feedback. *Studies in Educational Evaluation*, 39(3), 180–187. https://doi.org/10.1016/j.stueduc.2013.06.003

Hyland, K. (2014). Re-imagining literacy: English in Hong Kong's new university curriculum. In D. Coniam (Ed.), *English language education and assessment* (pp. 139–151). Singapore: Springer.

Hyland, K. (2016a). Writing with attitude: Conveying a stance in academic texts. In E. Hinkel (Ed.), *Teaching English grammar to speakers of other languages*. London: Routledge.

Hyland, K. (2016b). General and specific EAP. In K. Hyland & P. Shaw (Eds.), *The Routledge handbook of English for academic purposes* (pp. 41–53). London: Routledge.

Hyland, K., & Hamp-Lyons, L. (2002). EAP: Issues and directions. *Journal of English for Academic Purposes*, 1, 1–12. https://doi.org/10.1016/S1475-1585(02)00002-4

Hyland, K., & Jiang, F. (2016a). Change of attitude? A diachronic study of stance. *Written Communication*, 33(3), 251–274. https://doi.org/10.1177/0741088316650399

Hyland, K., & Jiang, F. K. (2016b). "We must conclude that …": A diachronic study of academic engagement. *Journal of English for Academic Purposes*, 24, 29–42. https://doi.org/10.1016/j.jeap.2016.09.003

Hyland, K., & Tse, P. (2004). Metadiscourse in academic writing: A reappraisal. *Applied Linguistics*, 25(2), 156–177. https://doi.org/10.1093/applin/25.2.156

Hyland, K., & Tse, P. (2009). Academic lexis and disciplinary practice: Corpus evidence for specificity. *International Journal of English Studies*, 9(2).

James, M. A. (2010). Transfer climate and EAP education: Students' perceptions of challenges to learning to transfer. *English for Specific Purposes*, 29, 133–147. https://doi.org/10.1016/j.esp.2009.09.002

James, M. A. (2012). An investigation of motivation to transfer second language learning. *The Modern Language Journal*, 96, 51–69. https://doi.org/10.1111/j.1540-4781.2012.01281.x

Jarvis, S., & Paquot, M. (2012). Exploring the role of n-grams in L1 identification. In S. Jarvis & S. Crossley (Eds.), *Approaching language transfer through text classification: Explorations in the detection-based approach* (pp. 71–105). Bristol: Multilingual Matters. https://doi.org/10.21832/9781847696991-004

Jensen, P. B., Jensen, L. J., & Brunak, S. (2012). Mining electronic health records: Towards better research applications and clinical care. *Nature Reviews Genetics*, 13(6), 395. https://doi.org/10.1038/nrg3208

Jiang, F. K., & Hyland, K. (2016). Nouns and academic interactions: A neglected feature of metadiscourse. *Applied Linguistics*, 39(4), 508–531.

Johns, T. (1991). Should you be persuaded – two examples of data-driven learning materials. In T. Johns, & P. King (Eds.), *Classroom concordancing. English Language Research Journal* (Vol. 4, pp. 1–16). Birmingham: Birmingham University.

Jurafsky, D., & Martin, J. (2009). *Speech and language processing: An introduction to natural language processing, computational linguistics, and speech recognition* (2nd ed.) Upper Saddle River, NJ: Prentice Hall.

Kaiser, H. F. (1960). The application of electronic computers to factor analysis. *Educational and psychological measurement*, 20(1), 141–151. https://doi.org/10.1177/001316446002000116

Kaufer, D., Geisler, C., Vlachos, P., & Ishizaki, S. (2006). Mining textual knowledge for writing education and research: The DocuScope project. In L. van Waes, M. Leijten & C. Neuwirth, (Eds.), *Writing and digital media* (pp. 115–129). Amsterdam: Elsevier.

Kaufer, D. S., Ishizaki, S., Butler, B. S., & Collins, J. (2004). *The power of words: Unveiling the speaker and writer's hidden craft*. London: Routledge.

Kessler, J. S. (2017). Scattertext: A browser-based tool for visualizing how corpora differ. *arXiv preprint* arXiv:1703.00565. https://doi.org/10.18653/v1/P17-4015

Kilgarriff, A., Rychly, P., Smrz, P., & Tugwell, D. (2004). The sketch engine. *Information Technology*, 105, 116.

Kilgarriff, A., & Grefenstette, G. (2003). Introduction to the special issue on web as corpus. *Computational Linguistics*, 29, 333–347. https://doi.org/10.1162/089120103322711569

Kostenko V. (2016). Language and cultural barriers in written communication in dentistry. *Akademia Pomorska w Slupsku*, 4, 238–249.

Kostenko, V. (2017). *Pragmatic and communicative aspects of case reports in dentistry* (Unpublished doctoral dissertation). Pomeranian University, Slupsk.

Kostenko, V. (2018). How to incorporate academic writing pedagogy in undergraduate and postgraduate medical education. *Wiadomości Lekarskie*, 2, 261–265.

Kunter, G. (2017). *Coquery* (version 0.10) [Computer Software]. Retrieved from <https://www.coquery.org/>

Kyle, K., & Crossley, S. A. (2015). Automatically assessing lexical sophistication: Indices, tools, findings, and application. *TESOL Quarterly*, 49(4), 757–786. https://doi.org/10.1002/tesq.194

Lakoff, G. (1972). Hedges: A study in meaning criteria and the logic of fuzzy concepts. *Chicago Linguistic Society Papers*, 8, 183–228.

Lancaster, Z. (2016). Expressing stance in undergraduate writing: Discipline-specific and general qualities. *Journal of English for Academic Purposes*, 23, 16–30. https://doi.org/10.1016/j.jeap.2016.05.006

Larsen-Freeman, D. (2011). A complexity theory approach to second language development / acquisition. In D. Atkinson (Ed.), *Alternative approaches to second language acquisition* (pp. 48–72). London: Routledge.

Lasswell, H. D., & Namenwirth, J. Z. (1969). *The Lasswell value dictionary*. New Haven, CT: New Haven.

Lave, J., & Wenger, E. (1991). *Situated learning: Legitimate peripheral participation*. Cambridge: Cambridge University Press. https://doi.org/10.1017/CBO9780511815355

Lee, D., & Swales, J. (2006). A corpus-based EAP course for NNS doctoral students: Moving from available specialized corpora to self-compiled corpora. *English for Specific Purposes*, 25, 56–75. https://doi.org/10.1016/j.esp.2005.02.010

Lee, H., Warschauer, M., & Lee, J. H. (2018). The effects of corpus use on second language vocabulary learning: A multilevel meta-analysis. *Applied Linguistics*, amy012. https://doi.org/10.1093/applin/amy012

Lee, J. J., Hitchcock, C., & Casal, J. E. (2018). Citation practices of L2 university students in first-year writing: Form, function, and stance. *Journal of English for Academic Purposes*, 33, 1–11. https://doi.org/10.1016/j.jeap.2018.01.001

Leech, G. (1997). Teaching and language corpora: A convergence. In A.Wichmann, S. Fligelstone, T. McEnery & G. Knowles (Eds.), *Teaching and language corpora* (pp. 1–23). London: Longman.

Lénko-Szymánska, A., & Boulton, A. (Eds.). (2015). *Multiple affordances of language corpora for data-driven learning*. Amsterdam: John Benjamins.

Leong, P. A. (2014). The passive voice in scientific writing. The current norm in science journals. *Journal of Science Communication*, 13(1), 1–16.

Lingard, L. (2015). Enlisting the power of the verb. *Perspectives on Medical Education*, 4(2), 53–54. https://doi.org/10.1007/s40037-015-0177-9

Lingard, L., Garwood, K., Schryer, C. F., & Spafford, M. M. (2003). A certain art of uncertainty: Case presentation and the development of professional identity. *Social Science & Medicine*, 56(3), 603–616. https://doi.org/10.1016/S0277-9536(02)00057-6

Liu, M., Calvo, R. A., & Rus, V. (2012). G-Asks: An intelligent automatic question generation system for academic writing support. *Dialogue & Discourse*, 3(2), 101–124. https://doi.org/10.5087/dad.2012.205

Lockwood, J. (2017). Towards a specific writing assessment at Hong Kong universities. In J. Flowerdew & T. Costley (Eds.), *Discipline-specific writing: Theory into practice* (pp. 196–215). London: Routledge.

Long, M. (1991). Focus on form: A design feature in language teaching methodology. In K. de Bot, R. Ginsberg, & C. Kramsch (Eds.) *Foreign language research in cross-cultural perspective.* Amsterdam: John Benjamins. https://doi.org/10.1075/sibil.2.07lon

Lu, X. (2010). Automatic analysis of syntactic complexity in second language writing. *International Journal of Corpus Linguistics*, 15(4), 474–496. https://doi.org/10.1075/ijcl.15.4.02lu

Luo, Q. (2016). The effects of data-driven learning activities on EFL learners' writing development. *SpringerPlus*, 5(1), 1255. https://doi.org/10.1186/s40064-016-2935-5

Manchón, R. M. (Ed.). (2011). *Learning-to-write and writing-to-learn in an additional language.* Amsterdam: John Benjamins. https://doi.org/10.1075/lllt.31

Martin, J. R., & White, P. R. (2003). *The language of evaluation* (Vol. 2). Houndmills: Palgrave Macmillan.

McGuire, W. J. (1984). Public communication as a strategy for inducing health-promoting behavioral change. *Preventive Medicine*, 13(3), 299–319. https://doi.org/10.1016/0091-7435(84)90086-0

Meurers, D. (2015). Learner corpora and natural language processing. In S. Granger, G. Gilquin, & F. Meunier (Eds.), *The Cambridge handbook of learner corpus research* (pp. 537–566). Cambridge: Cambridge University Press. https://doi.org/10.1017/CBO9781139649414.024

Millar, N. (2011). The processing of malformed formulaic language. *Applied Linguistics*, 32, 129–148. https://doi.org/10.1093/applin/amq035

Mischler, E. G. (1984). *The discourse of medicine: Dialectics of medical interviews.* Norwood, NJ: Ablex.

Mitton, C., Adair, C. E., McKenzie, E., Patten, S. B., & Waye Perry, B. (2007). Knowledge transfer and exchange: Review and synthesis of the literature. *Milbank Quarterly*, 85(4), 729–768. https://doi.org/10.1111/j.1468-0009.2007.00506.x

Molés-Cases, T., & Oster, U. (2015). Webquests in translator training. In A. Lénko-Szymánska & A. Boulton (Eds.), *Multiple affordances of language corpora for data-driven learning* (pp. 201–224). Amsterdam: John Benjamins.

Moretti, F. (2013). *Distant reading.* London: Verso Books.

Morrison, B. (2014). Challenges faced by non-native undergraduate student writers in an English-medium university. *The Asian ESP Journal*, 10(1), 136–174.

Morrison, B., & Evans, S. (2018). Supporting non-native speaker student writers making the transition from school to an English-medium university. *Language Learning in Higher Education*, 8(1), 1–20. https://doi.org/10.1515/cercles-2018-0001

Morse, Z., & Nakahara, S. (2001). English language education in Japanese dental schools. *European Journal of Dental Education*, 5(4), 168–172. https://doi.org/10.1034/j.1600-0579.2001.50405.x

Murakami, A. (2013). Cross-linguistic influence on the accuracy order of L2 English grammatical morphemes. In S. Granger, G. Gilquin, & F. Meunier (Eds.), *Twenty years of learner corpus research: Looking back, moving ahead.* (pp. 325–334). Louvain-la-Neuve: Presses Universitaires de Louvain.

Murakami, A., Thompson, P., Hunston, S., & Vajn, D. (2017). 'What is this corpus about?': Using topic modelling to explore a specialised corpus. *Corpora*, 12(2), 243–277. https://doi.org/10.3366/cor.2017.0118

Nadershahi, N., Bender, D. J., Lyon, C., & Blaseio, A (2013). An overview of case-based and problem-based learning methodologies for dental education. *Journal of Dental Education*, 77(10) 1300–1305.

Nesi, H. (2009). A multidimensional analysis of student writing across levels and disciplines. In M. Edwardes (Ed.), *Proceedings of the BAAL annual conference 2008: 41st annual meeting of the British Association for Applied Linguistics, 11–13 September 2008: Taking the measure of applied linguistics, Swansea University* (pp. 11–13). London: Scitsiugnil Press

Nesi, H., & Gardner, S. (2012). *Genres across the disciplines: Student writing in higher education.* Cambridge: Cambridge University Press.

Newell, G. E. (2008). Writing to learn: How alternative theories of school writing account for student performance. In C. MacArthur, S. Graham, & J. Fitzgerald (Eds.), *Handbook of writing research* (pp. 235–247). London: Guilford Press.

Nini, A. (2015a). Multidimensional Analysis Tagger (Version 1.3) [Computer Doftware]. Retrieved from <https://sites.google.com/site/multidimensionaltagger/home>

Nini, A. (2015b). MAT Manual. Retrieved from <https://sites.google.com/site/multidimen sionaltagger/home>

O'Donnell, M. (2008). The UAM CorpusTool: Software for corpus annotation and exploration. In *Proceedings of the XXVI Congreso de AESLA, Almeria, Spain, 3–5 April* (pp. 3–5).

Ott, N., & Meurers, D. (2010). Information retrieval for education: Making search engines language aware. *Themes in Science and Technology Education*, 3(1–2), 109–143.

Pak, A., & Paroubek, P. (2010, May). Twitter as a corpus for sentiment analysis and opinion mining. In *LREC* (Vol. 10, No. 2010).

Pang, B., & Lee, L. (2008). Opinion mining and sentiment analysis. *Foundations and Trends in Information Retrieval*, 2(1–2), 1–135. https://doi.org/10.1561/1500000011

Parkinson, J., Demecheleer, M., & Mackay, J. (2017). Writing like a builder: Acquiring a professional genre in a pedagogical setting. *English for Specific Purposes*, 46, 29–44. https://doi.org/10.1016/j.esp.2016.12.003

Pendar, N., & Chappelle, C. (2008). Investigating the promise of learner corpora: Methodological issues. *Calico Journal*, 25(2), 189–206.

Pérez-Paredes, P., Sánchez-Tornel, M., Alcaraz Calero, J. M., & Jiménez, P. A. (2011). Tracking learners' actual uses of corpora: Guided vs non-guided corpus consultation. *Computer Assisted Language Learning*, 24(3), 233–253. https://doi.org/10.1080/09588221.2010.539978

Polio, C. & Park, J. H. (2016). Language development in second language writing. In R. M. Manchón & P. K. Matsuda (Eds.), *Handbook of second and foreign language writing* (pp. 287–306). Berlin: De Gruyter. https://doi.org/10.1515/9781614511335-016

Poon, A. (2010). Language use, and language policy and planning in Hong Kong. *Current Issues in Language Planning*, 11, 1–66. https://doi.org/10.1080/14664201003682327

Quinn, C. (2014). Training L2 writers to reference corpora as a self-correction tool. *ELT Journal*, 69(2), 165–177. https://doi.org/10.1093/elt/ccu062

Rayson, P. (2016). *Log-likelihood calculator* [Computer Software]. Retrieved from <http://ucrel.lancs.ac.uk/llwizard.html>

Rayson, P. (2008). From key words to key semantic domains. *International Journal of Corpus Linguistics*, 13(4), 519–549. https://doi.org/10.1075/ijcl.13.4.06ray

Rayson, P. (2009). *Wmatrix: A web-based corpus processing environment* [Computer Software]. Lancaster: University of Lancaster.

Rayson, P., Archer, D., Piao, S., & McEnery, A. M. (2004). *The UCREL semantic analysis system* [Computer Software]. Lancaster: University of Lancaster.

Rayson, P., & Garside, R. (1998). The CLAWS web tagger. *ICAME Journal*, 22, 121–123.

Richards, P. S., & Inglehart, M. R. (2006). An interdisciplinary approach to case-based teaching: Does it create patient-centered and culturally sensitive providers? *Journal of Dental Education*, 70(3), 284–291.

Riley, K. (1991). Passive voice and rhetorical role in scientific writing. *Journal of Technical Writing and Communication*, 21(3), 239–257. https://doi.org/10.2190/Y51Y-P6QF-3LCC-4AUH

Römer, U. (2011). Corpus research applications in second language teaching. *Annual Review of Applied Linguistics*, 31, 205–225. https://doi.org/10.1017/S0267190511000055

Römer, U., & Swales, J. M. (2010). The Michigan corpus of upper-level student papers (MICUSP) [Computer Software]. Retrieved from <http://micusp.elicorpora.info/> https://doi.org/10.1016/j.jeap.2010.04.002

Salager-Meyer, F. (1991). Hedging in medical discourse: 1980-1990. *Interface*, 6(1), 33–54.

Salager-Meyer, F. (1994). Hedges and textual communicative function in medical English written discourse. *English for Specific Purposes*, 13(2), 149–170. https://doi.org/10.1016/0889-4906(94)90013-2

Schmidt, R. (1990). The role of consciousness in second language learning. *Applied Linguistics*, 11(2), 129–158. https://doi.org/10.1093/applin/11.2.129

Schryer, C. F., Lingard, L., Spafford, M., & Garwood, K. (2003). Structure and agency in medical case presentations. In C. Bazerman & D. Russell (Eds.), *Writing selves/writing societies: Research from activity perspectives* (pp. 62–96). Fort Collins, CO: The WAC Clearinghouse and Mind, Culture, and Activity.

Schryer, C. F., Lingard, L., & Spafford, M. (2007). Regularised practices: Genres, improvisation, and identity formation in health-care professions. In M. Zachry & C. Thralls (Eds.), *Communicative practices in workplaces and the professions: Cultural perspectives on the regulation of discourse and organizations* (pp. 21–44). London: Routledge.

Schubert, C. (2016). Current trends in register research. In C. Schubert & C. Sanchez-Stockhammer (Eds.), *Variational text linguistics: Revisiting register in English* (pp. 1–18). Berlin: De Gruyter. https://doi.org/10.1515/9783110443554-002

Simsek, D., Shum, S. B., De Liddo, A., Ferguson, R., & Sándor, Á. (2014, March). Visual analytics of academic writing. In *Proceedings of the Fourth International Conference on Learning Analytics and Knowledge* (pp. 265–266). ACM. https://doi.org/10.1145/2567574.2567577

Sinclair, J. (1991). *Corpus, concordance and collocation*. Oxford: Oxford University Press.

Sinclair, J. (1999). A way with common words. In H. Hasselgard & S. Oksefjell (Eds.), *Out of corpora: Studies in honour of Stig Johansson* (pp. 157–159). Amsterdam: Rodopi.

Small, H. (2011). Interpreting maps of science using citation context sentiments: A preliminary investigation. *Scientometrics*, 87(2), 373–388. https://doi.org/10.1007/s11192-011-0349-2

Stone, P., Dunphy, D. C., Smith, M. S., & Ogilvie, D. M. (1968). The general inquirer: A computer approach to content analysis. *Journal of Regional Science*, 8(1), 113–116.

Swales, J. (1990). *Genre analysis: English in academic and research settings*. Cambridge: Cambridge University Press.

Swales, J. (2014). Variation in citational practice in a corpus of student biology papers: From parenthetical plonking to intertextual storytelling. *Written Communication*, 31, 118–141. https://doi.org/10.1177/0741088313515166

Swales, J., & Burke, A. (2003). It's really fascinating work: Differences in evaluative adjectives across academic registers. In P. Leistyna, & C. Meyer (Eds.), *Corpus analysis. Language structure and language use* (pp. 1–18). Amsterdam: Rodopi.

Swales, J., & Feak, C. (2000). *English in today's research world.* Ann Arbor, MI: University of Michigan Press. https://doi.org/10.3998/mpub.9059

The BNC Sampler. (1999). Oxford, UK: Oxford University Computing Services.

Thomas, J. (2015). Stealing a march on collocation: Deriving extended collocations from full-text for student analysis and synthesis. In In A. Lénko-Szymánska & A. Boulton (Eds.), *Multiple affordances of language corpora for data-driven learning* (pp. 85–108). Amsterdam: John Benjamins.

Tono, Y., Satake, Y., & Miura, A. (2014). The effects of using corpora on revision tasks in L2 writing with coded error feedback. *ReCALL*, 26, 147–162. https://doi.org/10.1017/S095834401400007X

Toutanova, K., Klein, D., Manning, C. D., & Singer, Y. (2003, May). Feature-rich part-of-speech tagging with a cyclic dependency network. *In Proceedings of the 2003 Conference of the North American Chapter of the Association for Computational Linguistics on Human Language Technology* (Vol. 1, pp. 173–180). Stroudsburg, PA: Association for Computational Linguistics.

Tribble, C. (2001). Small corpora and teaching writing. In M. Ghadessy, A. Henry, & R. L. Roseberry (Eds.), *Small corpus studies and ELT: Theory and practice* (pp. 381–408). Amsterdam: John Benjamins. https://doi.org/10.1075/scl.5.22tri

Tribble, C., & Wingate, U. (2013). From text to corpus: A genre-based approach to academic literacy instruction. *System*, 41, 307–321. https://doi.org/10.1016/j.system.2013.03.001

Trudgill, P. (2000). *Sociolinguistics: An introduction to language and society* (4th edn). London: Penguin.

Whiteside, K. & Wharton, S. (2019). Semantic patterning of grammatical keywords in undergraduate academic writing from two close disciplines. *Journal of English for Academic Purposes*, 39, 1–20.

Widdowson, H. G. (1998). Context, community, and authentic language. *TESOL Quarterly*, 32(4), 705–716. https://doi.org/10.2307/3588001

Widmann, J., Koh, K., & Ziai, R. (2011). The SACODEYL search tool: Exploiting corpora for language learning purposes. In A. Frankenberg-Garcia, L. Flowerdew, & G. Aston (Eds.), *New trends in corpora and language learning* (pp. 167–178). London: Continuum.

Williams, G. (2012). Bringing data and dictionary together: Real science in real dictionaries. In A. Boulton, Carter-Thomas, S., & Rowley-Jolivet, E. (Eds.), *Corpus-informed research and learning in ESP: Issues and applications* (pp. 217–238). Amsterdam: John Benjamins. https://doi.org/10.1075/scl.52.09wil

Williams, I. A. (1996). A contextual study of lexical verbs in two types of medical research report: Clinical and experimental. *English for Specific Purposes*, 15, 175–197. https://doi.org/10.1016/0889-4906(96)00010-5

Wilson, A. (2013). Embracing Bayes factors for key item analysis in corpus linguistics. In M. Bieswanger & A. Koll-Stobbe (Eds.), *New approaches to the study of linguistic variability* (pp. 3–11). Frankfurt: Peter Lang.

Winker, M. A. (2006). Clinical Crossroads: Expanding the horizons. *JAMA*, 295(24), 2888–2888. https://doi.org/10.1001/jama.295.24.2888

Wu, H., & Badger, R. G. (2009). In a strange and uncharted land: ESP teachers' strategies for dealing with unpredicted problems in subject knowledge during class. *English for Specific Purposes*, 28(1), 19–32. https://doi.org/10.1016/j.esp.2008.09.003

Wu, J. C., Chang, Y. C., Mitamura, T., & Chang, J. S. (2010, July). Automatic collocation suggestion in academic writing. In *Proceedings of the ACL 2010 Conference Short Papers* (pp. 115–119). Stroudsburg, PA: Association for Computational Linguistics.

Yan, E., Williams, J., Chen, Z. (2017). Understanding disciplinary vocabularies using a full-text enabled domain-independent term extraction approach. *PLoS ONE* 12(11): e0187762. https://doi.org/10.1371/journal.pone.0187762

Yoon, H. (2008). More than a linguistic reference: The influence of corpus technology on L2 academic writing. *Language Learning & Technology*, 12, 31–49 19-32.

Yoon, H., & Hirvela, A. (2004). ESL student attitude toward corpus use in L2 writing. *Journal of Second Language Writing*, 13, 257–283. https://doi.org/10.1016/j.jslw.2004.06.002

Young, S. S., & Karr, A. (2011). Deming, data and observational studies. *Significance*, 8, 116–120. https://doi.org/10.1111/j.1740-9713.2011.00506.x

Yu, B., & Zhang, F. (2015). Disciplinary difference in citation opinion expressions. *iConference 2015 Proceedings*.

Appendix A. Language Features in EFA Model (Chapter 2)

	Factor loadings					
	Factor 1	Factor 2	Factor 3	Factor 4	Factor 5	Uniqueness
ANDC	.	.	.	.	.	0.686
BEMA	.	.	.	.	.	0.746
BYPA	.	.	.	.	.	0.849
CC	.	.	.	.	0.449	0.685
COND	0.475	.	.	.	.	0.721
DEMP	0.644	.	.	.	.	0.569
EX	.	.	.	.	.	0.728
GER	.	.	.	.	.	0.708
HDG	.	.	.	.	.	0.980
INPR	.	.	.	.	.	0.900
JJ	.	.	.	.	−0.566	0.562
NN	.	.	.	.	−0.466	0.544
OSUB	.	.	.	.	.	0.874
PASS	.	.	.	0.94	.	0.101
PEAS	.	.	.	.	0.593	0.557
PLACE	.	.	.	.	.	0.781
POS	.	.	.	.	.	0.974
PRMD	0.751	.	.	.	.	0.438
PROD	.	.	0.408	.	.	0.800
PRP	.	.	.	.	.	0.917
QUPR	.	.	.	.	.	0.856
RP	.	.	.	.	.	0.787
SMP	.	.	.	.	.	0.907
SPP2	.	0.419	.	.	.	0.814
SUAV	.	.	.	.	.	0.797
SYM	.	.	.	.	.	0.723
THAC	.	.	.	.	.	0.870
THVC	.	.	.	.	.	0.808
TIME	.	.	.	.	.	0.929
TPP3	.	.	.	−0.460	.	0.535
VB	0.686	.	.	.	.	0.365
VBD	.	.	0.815	.	.	0.268
VBN	.	.	.	0.854	.	0.235
VPRT	.	.	−0.815	.	.	0.165
WDT	.	.	−0.477	.	.	0.756
WHCL	0.423	.	.	.	.	0.746
WHOBJ	.	.	.	.	.	0.891
WHQU	.	.	.	.	.	0.847
WHSUB	.	0.890	.	.	.	0.223
WP	.	0.924	.	.	.	0.087
WZPRES	.	.	.	.	.	0.869

Appendix B. Keywords from the dentistry research article corpus (Chapter 2)

Word	Freq. in dentistry corpus	LL	Word	Freq. in dentistry corpus	LL
dental	1165	2089.468	macrodontia	17	31.901
teeth	721	1298.185	microtensile	17	31.901
tooth	699	1240.112	odontoblasts	17	31.901
caries	586	1064.953	overdentures	17	31.901
periodontal	386	711.414	paste	17	31.901
dentin	373	699.94	pit	17	31.901
enamel	336	607.987	stump	17	31.901
oral	541	578.879	fissure	17	31.901
resin	324	553.97	reason	67	31.656
restorations	261	489.771	provision	31	31.33
implant	305	487.774	service	83	31.271
materials	305	471.329	bur	23	31.207
etch	253	462.681	calibrated	23	31.207
surface	379	448.68	epinephrine	23	31.207
dentine	223	418.463	phenyl	23	31.207
ceramic	246	404.544	solutions	34	30.844
crowns	214	401.574	increment	25	30.824
adhesive	209	371.562	standards	25	30.824
bone	428	367.346	dren	27	30.796
material	273	365.359	stabilization	27	30.796
periodontitis	194	364.044	anova	48	30.599
bond	212	337.032	acrylic	20	30.483
implants	211	335.23	answers	20	30.483
specimens	263	282.015	radiographs	41	30.236
restorative	154	277.896	clinics	61	30.125
molars	146	273.971	evaluated	96	30.044
bonding	146	262.99	adipocytes	16	30.024
surfaces	161	256.38	apposition	16	30.024
wear	148	251.251	bioengineered	16	30.024
maxillary	143	242.072	buehler	16	30.024
occlusal	129	242.07	ethane	16	30.024
mandibular	131	235.058	kuraray	16	30.024
zirconia	131	235.058	lactobacilli	16	30.024
restoration	156	227.092	mesio	16	30.024
composite	205	225.854	microspectroscopy	16	30.024
strength	203	225.669	ovation	16	30.024
orthodontic	116	217.676	streptococci	16	30.024
fracture	230	216.043	table	512	29.863

Word	Freq. in dentistry corpus	LL	Word	Freq. in dentistry corpus	LL
bracket	115	215.799	variances	22	29.501
crown	114	213.923	significant	155	29.413
adhesives	112	210.17	examinations	47	29.365
wire	117	209.012	micro	43	29.277
incisal	110	206.417	thermal	26	29.2
width	129	204.34	tip	26	29.2
rinse	106	198.911	tested	126	28.757
shade	106	198.911	ceased	19	28.706
force	176	197.899	foreign	19	28.706
denture	103	193.281	lidocaine	19	28.706
dentition	102	191.405	sites	125	28.7
hypodontia	102	191.405	purpose	55	28.657
color	113	187.173	electron	34	28.617
dentistry	99	185.775	cementum	15	28.148
slot	99	185.775	chlorhexidine	15	28.148
veneers	99	185.775	cleansing	15	28.148
ridge	103	182.995	commission	15	28.148
sedation	110	181.703	dentifrice	15	28.148
permanent	125	177.508	endodontically	15	28.148
properties	184	172.351	erupted	15	28.148
habits	132	169.341	gingivalis	15	28.148
pulp	89	167.01	grinding	15	28.148
dentists	93	164.433	guides	15	28.148
sucking	87	163.257	healed	15	28.148
stress	215	162.635	ionomer	15	28.148
bulk	96	162.605	juices	15	28.148
technique	142	162.078	luting	15	28.148
layer	113	161.069	microbial	15	28.148
molar	97	158.052	nanocomposite	15	28.148
dentures	83	155.751	object	15	28.148
composites	81	151.998	rounded	15	28.148
hydroxyapatite	81	151.998	sticks	15	28.148
etching	80	150.121	sugar	15	28.148
root	122	149.176	wax	15	28.148
chewing	79	148.245	distal	46	28.143
attachment	94	146.94	partially	38	28.114
hybrid	99	145.736	academic	35	27.933
acid	167	145.358	morphological	27	27.893
arch	81	142.189	gestational	21	27.802
application	146	138.049	scaffolds	21	27.802
universal	106	136.886	paper	53	27.736

Word	Freq. in dentistry corpus	LL	Word	Freq. in dentistry corpus	LL
marginal	85	136.314	specialist	25	27.615
extraction	112	136.164	canal	23	27.542
present	334	134.338	condition	64	27.331
light	138	133.568	movement	33	27.216
brackets	71	133.233	question	68	26.993
cusp	71	133.233	training	68	26.993
dentist	71	133.233	engineering	18	26.935
lingual	71	133.233	replacing	18	26.935
premolar	71	133.233	royal	18	26.935
veneer	71	133.233	scaffold	18	26.935
hardness	70	131.356	measuring	45	26.933
cement	68	127.603	bindings	14	26.271
buccal	73	127.384	butt	14	26.271
behaviour	119	125.797	cavitation	14	26.271
gingival	67	125.727	collagenolytic	14	26.271
ection	79	125.486	colonization	14	26.271
values	294	124.642	dentsply	14	26.271
mechanical	149	122.129	drying	14	26.271
abrasion	65	121.973	endarterectomy	14	26.271
fill	64	120.097	fees	14	26.271
modulus	93	118.806	jig	14	26.271
phosphoric	63	118.22	kruskal	14	26.271
posts	63	118.22	mastication	14	26.271
prosthetic	68	118.142	microfill	14	26.271
repaired	68	118.142	mineralization	14	26.271
load	175	117.529	operators	14	26.271
incisors	62	116.344	osteon	14	26.271
mode	114	115.383	periapical	14	26.271
fluoride	65	112.602	polymer	14	26.271
depth	99	108.883	prosthodontic	14	26.271
step	130	108.169	silanes	14	26.271
friction	57	106.961	stubs	14	26.271
water	193	104.255	subgingival	14	26.271
impression	69	102.441	tabs	14	26.271
wet	59	101.535	theme	14	26.271
subjects	235	101.309	viscoelastic	14	26.271
placement	82	100.548	wallis	14	26.271
edentulous	53	99.455	wings	14	26.271
vertical	53	99.455	fissures	14	26.271
bonded	52	97.579	trait	20	26.112
brushing	51	95.702	device	24	26.041

Word	Freq. in dentistry corpus	LL	Word	Freq. in dentistry corpus	LL
schools	81	95.565	pathogens	43	26.04
dry	72	94.769	increments	22	25.916
specimen	93	93.989	environment	49	25.897
incisor	50	93.826	unaffected	32	25.829
premolars	50	93.826	adjacent	45	25.459
mandible	58	93.286	cavities	17	25.17
problems	110	92.836	contract	17	25.17
amalgam	49	91.949	nitrous	17	25.17
canines	49	91.949	commercial	30	25.125
interface	72	91.039	irradiation	30	25.125
bite	53	90.489	seconds	30	25.125
torque	48	90.073	sectioned	30	25.125
school	119	89.126	adolescents	42	24.837
placed	120	88.586	young	83	24.772
preventive	83	86.76	success	49	24.577
maximum	117	86.464	concluded	31	24.455
cervical	73	85.846	guidance	31	24.455
loading	95	84.693	biomechanical	19	24.431
saliva	45	84.443	compressive	19	24.431
silane	45	84.443	consultant	19	24.431
toothbrushing	45	84.443	max	19	24.431
indentation	53	84.258	paediatric	19	24.431
elastic	72	84.228	bisphosphonate	13	24.395
dimensions	65	82.997	bifidobacteria	13	24.395
mesial	44	82.567	demineralised	13	24.395
chemical	64	81.326	dentitions	13	24.395
translucency	48	81.303	dentogingival	13	24.395
silica	43	80.69	desmoplastic	13	24.395
widths	43	80.69	disturbances	13	24.395
applied	183	80.678	ections	13	24.395
cavity	59	80.586	fillers	13	24.395
hard	50	78.857	hyperdontia	13	24.395
ferrule	42	78.814	hypochlorite	13	24.395
thickness	105	77.979	interceptive	13	24.395
hygiene	57	77.163	microhardness	13	24.395
etched	41	76.937	nanomechanical	13	24.395
toothbrush	41	76.937	osteoporosis	13	24.395
self	247	76.881	probiotic	13	24.395
loads	59	76.652	sealing	13	24.395
failures	45	75.801	simulate	13	24.395
facial	79	75.471	sounding	13	24.395

Word	Freq. in dentistry corpus	LL	Word	Freq. in dentistry corpus	LL
natural	124	75.129	tags	13	24.395
monomers	40	75.061	tetric	13	24.395
tensile	40	75.061	triethoxysilyl	13	24.395
maxilla	44	73.969	unsupported	13	24.395
pellet	50	73.747	voco	13	24.395
osteons	39	73.184	wearing	13	24.395
prenatal	39	73.184	woven	13	24.395
sealants	39	73.184	variables	143	24.335
twin	39	73.184	transverse	21	24.301
resistance	132	72.882	mothers	44	24.294
distance	72	72.595	removal	44	24.294
referral	68	71.884	intact	35	24.191
filler	38	71.308	osseous	26	23.862
nanoleakage	38	71.308	sound	26	23.862
pneumoniae	38	71.308	peak	76	23.858
smokeless	38	71.308	gap	46	23.847
unloading	38	71.308	parameters	54	23.844
repair	97	71.083	apple	16	23.411
vita	42	70.308	chemically	16	23.411
smear	48	70.232	cleaned	16	23.411
bacteria	55	69.947	depths	16	23.411
particles	55	69.947	infiltration	16	23.411
cuspal	37	69.431	osteoblasts	16	23.411
probing	37	69.431	property	16	23.411
juice	47	68.478	significant	232	23.257
speed	54	68.279	experimental	74	22.977
matrix	74	68.096	clinic	73	22.974
educational	60	68.092	reasons	73	22.974
mouth	56	68.082	master	22	22.93
approximal	36	67.555	film	20	22.697
resorption	36	67.555	degradation	31	22.547
stresses	51	66.968	aesthetics	12	22.518
collagen	91	66.838	appliances	12	22.518
displacement	40	66.651	asperger	12	22.518
dimension	53	66.615	backings	12	22.518
restored	76	66.404	cleaning	12	22.518
longevity	43	66.312	epoxy	12	22.518
ceramics	35	65.678	graduating	12	22.518
porcelain	35	65.678	intraoral	12	22.518
height	90	65.518	mcgill	12	22.518
horizontal	39	64.824	osteonecrosis	12	22.518

Word	Freq. in dentistry corpus	LL	Word	Freq. in dentistry corpus	LL
talon	39	64.824	rinsing	12	22.518
thick	56	64.801	tariffs	12	22.518
alendronate	34	63.802	topography	12	22.518
demineralization	34	63.802	alloy	57	22.471
filtek	34	63.802	stability	40	22.471
masticatory	34	63.802	abstract	133	22.372
monomer	34	63.802	stem	82	22.295
steel	34	63.802	management	95	22.121
supernumerary	34	63.802	soft	69	22.092
twins	34	63.802	accepted	32	22.068
attachments	38	62.999	appearance	32	22.068
preparation	82	62.357	england	32	22.068
conclusion	125	62.276	filled	23	21.848
tissues	94	61.963	indicators	23	21.848
articaine	33	61.925	statistical	138	21.699
cherubism	33	61.925	dentate	15	21.659
deformation	33	61.925	fractured	15	21.659
scotchbond	33	61.925	nova	15	21.659
machine	43	61.489	rectangular	15	21.659
strain	79	60.239	triglycerides	15	21.659
canine	70	60.06	fee	21	21.395
fabricated	32	60.048	post	126	21.225
peri	49	59.999	extracted	47	21.185
experience	99	58.651	biologic	19	21.107
titanium	72	58.627	graft	19	21.107
techniques	90	58.59	thermo	19	21.107
examiners	31	58.172	topical	19	21.107
diamond	41	58.012	immersed	17	21.1
interdisciplinary	35	57.532	modified	27	20.981
glass	55	57.325	introduction	150	20.716
mucosa	43	57.301	presented	94	20.68
esthetic	30	56.295	accordance	36	20.657
sealant	30	56.295	abrasive	11	20.642
formation	70	55.867	adhering	11	20.642
margins	34	55.713	aluminum	11	20.642
layers	37	55.64	atheromas	11	20.642
japan	59	55.62	brasseler	11	20.642
reported	488	55.098	cementation	11	20.642
curing	29	54.419	cemento	11	20.642
mineralized	29	54.419	cementoblasts	11	20.642
showed	252	54.11	clearfil	11	20.642

Word	Freq. in dentistry corpus	LL	Word	Freq. in dentistry corpus	LL
shape	51	53.913	clip	11	20.642
thin	41	53.912	commissioning	11	20.642
jaw	33	53.895	crestal	11	20.642
tubules	33	53.895	crosshead	11	20.642
mucosal	47	53.493	dimethacrylate	11	20.642
archwire	28	52.542	disclosed	11	20.642
biotype	28	52.542	evaluators	11	20.642
chamfer	28	52.542	finish	11	20.642
debt	28	52.542	gala	11	20.642
nonnutritive	28	52.542	grandio	11	20.642
polished	28	52.542	holder	11	20.642
putty	28	52.542	hydrolytic	11	20.642
swedish	28	52.542	inorganic	11	20.642
fiber	50	52.365	numbness	11	20.642
wash	40	52.224	outreach	11	20.642
edentulism	35	52.103	panoramic	11	20.642
gold	44	51.832	prosthodontics	11	20.642
conventional	100	51.38	reinforcement	11	20.642
bending	27	50.666	reject	11	20.642
interproximal	27	50.666	shapes	11	20.642
roughness	27	50.666	sweets	11	20.642
particle	34	50.339	teach	11	20.642
ball	31	50.265	toothache	11	20.642
recorded	119	49.947	vivadent	11	20.642
gestation	36	49.38	fibrous	11	20.642
polymerization	36	49.38	partial	53	20.637
shaped	38	48.862	lateral	54	20.578
variance	59	48.85	replacement	37	20.397
albicans	26	48.789	failed	44	20.39
indenter	26	48.789	value	129	20.377
maxillofacial	26	48.789	autism	22	20.373
polishing	26	48.789	situations	25	20.243
salivary	26	48.789	questions	84	20.115
sharps	26	48.789	rated	33	20.056
filled	26	48.789	conventionally	14	19.916
procedures	121	48.69	dysplasia	14	19.916
radiographic	51	48.659	labial	14	19.916
difficulty	42	48.601	manufacturing	14	19.916
preservation	42	48.601	silicon	14	19.916
correlations	33	48.579	attend	20	19.875
gender	74	48.393	shortened	20	19.875

Word	Freq. in dentistry corpus	LL	Word	Freq. in dentistry corpus	LL
removed	67	48.027	highest	98	19.634
contact	99	47.716	suitable	26	19.632
found	357	47.682	referred	53	19.616
preterm	68	47.549	compression	23	19.548
healing	58	47.457	appointment	18	19.531
fit	45	47.406	direction	35	19.485
carious	25	46.913	respondents	66	19.475
stainless	25	46.913	inferior	16	19.452
yogurt	25	46.913	interfaces	16	19.452
impacted	32	46.821	prime	16	19.452
forces	56	46.759	experiences	36	19.248
bacterial	48	46.677	chosen	44	19.216
filler	29	46.643	teaching	31	19.168
habit	54	46.083	create	21	18.915
organic	34	45.956	referrals	21	18.915
bud	36	45.519	clearly	48	18.868
impacts	36	45.519	reference	129	18.801
aim	47	45.183	actinomycetemcomitans	10	18.765
penetration	31	45.068	amputated	10	18.765
ameloblastoma	24	45.036	analgesia	10	18.765
appointments	24	45.036	autopolymerizing	10	18.765
endodontic	24	45.036	brushed	10	18.765
esthetics	24	45.036	cariogenic	10	18.765
examiner	24	45.036	cavitated	10	18.765
featherstone	24	45.036	chipping	10	18.765
overjet	24	45.036	curettage	10	18.765
plasticine	24	45.036	effervescent	10	18.765
powder	24	45.036	exural	10	18.765
seas	24	45.036	forsythus	10	18.765
silver	24	45.036	giant	10	18.765
practitioners	70	45.027	grape	10	18.765
palatal	120	44.602	histomorphometric	10	18.765
edge	43	44.321	hybrids	10	18.765
method	153	43.49	infiltrated	10	18.765
core	55	43.324	instron	10	18.765
stiffness	30	43.319	intermedia	10	18.765
contracts	23	43.16	lightness	10	18.765
dentinal	23	43.16	mandatory	10	18.765
fabrication	23	43.16	nakashima	10	18.765
pacifier	23	43.16	niques	10	18.765
repairs	23	43.16	odontogenic	10	18.765

Word	Freq. in dentistry corpus	LL	Word	Freq. in dentistry corpus	LL
varnish	23	43.16	preschool	10	18.765
walls	23	43.16	pylori	10	18.765
shear	27	43.031	quitting	10	18.765
socio	42	42.79	redness	10	18.765
visual	47	42.774	regimes	10	18.765
examination	119	42.663	rods	10	18.765
retention	73	42.497	siloxane	10	18.765
plaque	40	42.45	spaces	10	18.765
measurements	116	41.793	speciality	10	18.765
mean	329	41.734	temporomandibular	10	18.765
crest	29	41.573	tolerances	10	18.765
lithium	29	41.573	toothpaste	10	18.765
abutment	22	41.283	toughness	10	18.765
aesthetic	22	41.283	trapezoidal	10	18.765
fibrils	22	41.283	visually	10	18.765
heritability	22	41.283	wing	10	18.765
isobmi	22	41.283	occurs	50	18.752
microleakage	22	41.283	posterior	84	18.712
removable	22	41.283	correlation	59	18.556
stone	22	41.283	measurement	59	18.556
veneered	22	41.283	study	1027	18.538
equation	41	41.266	carefully	25	18.301
artificial	26	41.228	embedded	25	18.301
interfacial	26	41.228	statement	25	18.301
margin	26	41.228	blends	13	18.183
provisional	26	41.228	oil	13	18.183
uncooperative	31	40.857	relating	13	18.183
authors	75	40.556	seizure	13	18.183
fear	35	40.501	translucent	13	18.183
deviations	28	39.832	unlabeled	22	18.144
prostheses	28	39.832	local	115	18.082
families	48	39.778	bipolar	17	17.971
medicaid	48	39.778	replaced	30	17.955
strains	48	39.778	corners	15	17.818
acidic	25	39.429	mixing	15	17.818
alumina	21	39.407	optical	15	17.818
decayed	21	39.407	reflection	15	17.818
disinfection	21	39.407	investigated	63	17.764
gloss	21	39.407	advice	31	17.667
ligating	21	39.407	pediatric	31	17.667
microorganisms	21	39.407	substrate	23	17.514

Word	Freq. in dentistry corpus	LL	Word	Freq. in dentistry corpus	LL
microwave	21	39.407	testing	141	17.488
mutans	21	39.407	microscope	32	17.415
oblique	21	39.407	structures	34	17.001
papilla	21	39.407	anchorage	9	16.889
polymerized	21	39.407	apatite	9	16.889
silicone	21	39.407	bitewing	9	16.889
spectrophotometer	21	39.407	bluff	9	16.889
spectrophotometric	21	39.407	cloth	9	16.889
thermocycling	21	39.407	crack	9	16.889
veneering	21	39.407	cycled	9	16.889
dried	30	39.168	deliveries	9	16.889
means	92	39.148	denuded	9	16.889
education	129	38.911	dibular	9	16.889
shrinkage	32	38.904	disilicate	9	16.889
parents	154	38.834	dome	9	16.889
missing	101	38.47	evoceram	9	16.889
lesions	80	38.295	finishing	9	16.889
revealed	119	37.998	fungi	9	16.889
cohesive	24	37.632	futurabond	9	16.889
sea	24	37.632	gum	9	16.889
clinical	461	37.541	hydrophilic	9	16.889
abutments	20	37.53	incrementally	9	16.889
anaesthetic	20	37.53	indents	9	16.889
myofascial	20	37.53	interabutment	9	16.889
reflectance	20	37.53	layering	9	16.889
socket	20	37.53	leukoplakia	9	16.889
made	150	37.17	luminescence	9	16.889
literature	80	37.073	mesh	9	16.889
bottom	43	37.019	mitutoyo	9	16.889
storage	38	36.743	orthodontists	9	16.889
one	526	36.654	predental	9	16.889
lesion	54	36.489	pulpal	9	16.889
anaesthesia	26	36.365	repairing	9	16.889
spectra	26	36.365	retainers	9	16.889
tokyo	26	36.365	retentive	9	16.889
mother	36	36.298	slide	9	16.889
oxide	59	36.231	snuff	9	16.889
demineralized	23	35.839	staic	9	16.889
eruption	23	35.839	substrates	9	16.889
quartz	23	35.839	sulcus	9	16.889
general	182	35.742	superelastic	9	16.889

Word	Freq. in dentistry corpus	LL	Word	Freq. in dentistry corpus	LL
backing	19	35.654	thoroughly	9	16.889
burs	19	35.654	trephine	9	16.889
cusps	19	35.654	unrestored	9	16.889
distilled	19	35.654	victory	9	16.889
extractions	19	35.654	viscosity	9	16.889
grit	19	35.654	wettability	9	16.889
methacrylate	19	35.654	firing	9	16.889
procera	19	35.654	hand	60	16.879
remineralization	19	35.654	functional	93	16.806
shades	19	35.654	apical	21	16.76
supreme	19	35.654	according	163	16.58
swallowing	19	35.654	faces	12	16.46
mineral	30	35.637	lasting	12	16.46
procedure	99	35.559	radiographically	12	16.46
stated	37	35.254	reparative	12	16.46
prepared	77	35.085	multidisciplinary	16	16.429
protective	58	35.018	orange	16	16.429
former	35	34.781	wavelength	16	16.429
remodelling	25	34.64	affect	67	16.372
conscious	27	34.14	desired	14	16.2
impressions	22	34.049	frameworks	14	16.2
jaws	22	34.049	placing	14	16.2
zirconium	22	34.049	rigid	14	16.2
carried	68	34.002	wore	14	16.2
artificial	18	33.777	cured	22	16.179
crossbite	18	33.777	sampling	43	16.066
gingivitis	18	33.777	check	19	16.055
irregular	18	33.777	profile	19	16.055
mold	18	33.777	calcium	33	15.905
nanoindentation	18	33.777	coronal	23	15.7
resins	18	33.777	suggested	78	15.679
roots	18	33.777	side	63	15.45
wall	46	33.163	discussion	201	15.426
nano	24	32.92	backgrounds	17	15.422
statistically	112	32.769	eye	17	15.422
covered	56	32.621	feedback	17	15.422
den	26	32.478	quartile	17	15.422
adhesion	28	32.401	angle	37	15.418
blend	21	32.264	pairs	37	15.418
guide	53	32.025	attached	20	15.397
cracks	17	31.901	designs	29	15.354

Word	Freq. in dentistry corpus	LL	Word	Freq. in dentistry corpus	LL
discoloration	17	31.901	retained	29	15.354
fill	17	31.901	situation	29	15.354
fissure	17	31.901	air	60	15.316
flexural	17	31.901	practitioner	24	15.299
grandioso	17	31.901	biological	40	15.205
ivoclar	17	31.901	diameter	40	15.205
			form	80	15.201
			differences	219	15.15

Index